CLEAN EATING

TABLE OF CONTENTS

CHAPTER ONE

CLEAN EATING: DEFINITION

What is Clean Eating?

Clean eating means eating foods as close to their original, natural state as possible. This means foods that do not have any artificial colors, flavors or preservatives. It also means avoiding foods that are overly processes or refined, are made with refined sugar and bleached flour, avoiding anything fried and avoiding drinks that are loaded with sugar. Basically, you eat the foods that our bodies evolved to eat and process.

Clean eating isn't really a diet. It's more of a lifestyle. This isn't something you do for a few months and then go back to processed, artificial foods. After eating clean for a while, you may actually find that these types of foods turn your stomach! Also, clean eating isn't about depriving yourself. It's about making smarter food choices. There are tons of great clean eating recipes that taste fabulous at the same time. You can even make cookies!

One key way to know if a food is clean is to determine if people have messed with it. That means adding things to improve the taste, color, shelf life etc. You want foods to be as close to their natural state as possible. When foods are altered with chemicals, colors, etc they lose their nutritional value. Clean food is low in salt, fat, sugar and additives. If the label has something in the ingredients that looks or sounds like a science project, that food is not clean. The cleanest foods are organic fruits and vegetables, but those are not your only options.

There are many benefits to eating clean. Not only will it help fight off or prevent numerous diseases, your energy levels will also increase. You'll also be able to deal with stress better and won't be on an emotional roller coaster. It boosts your metabolism so it can help you lose weight and then keep it off.

If you're trying to lose weight, the clean diet is a great way to do that. Since you're feeding your body what it is designed to use, it will react by losing weight if you need to. Part of eating clean also means not counting calories or feeling hungry. You eat small clean meals frequently to keep your metabolism revved up and combine a lean protein, complex carb and healthy fat into every meal. Also, your body will work more efficiently since it won't have to deal with all of the chemicals in processed foods.

Clean eating is a shift but is actually pretty easy to make. The results are quick and you'll start feeling better almost immediately. You'll also realize how many chemicals we put in our bodies just with the food we put in our mouths. It's pretty scary when you make that realization!

What Is Clean Eating and the Foods That Are Allowed?

Clean eating is one of the best ways to maintain or lose weight. But what exactly is clean eating or the foods that are allowed when eating clean. Clean eating is eating foods in there most natural form. So no processed, prepackaged meals that have added preservatives, sweeteners and sodium. Basically if it is in the form that God made it, then it is clean.

Here is a list to help get you started towards eating clean

Starchy Complex Carbs

Pick two to four servings of complex carbohydrates from starchy-carb sources or whole grains a day.

A serving size for each of these is the size of a cupped hand.

- Whole Grains

- Vegetable Sources
- Buckwheat
- Bananas
- Multi-Grain, buckwheat, Ezekiel, oat bran, and whole-meal spelt bread and wraps
- Carrots
- Oat-bran cereal
- Potatoes
- Oatmeal
- Radishes
- Quinoa
- Sweet Potatoes
- Spelt
- Yams
- Whole Barley
- Garbanzo beans (chick peas)
- Whole-wheat or brown rice couscous
- Kidney beans
- Whole-wheat, brown-rice or other whole-grain pasta
- Lentils
- Wild, black or brown rice
- Navy beans
- Pinto beans
- Soybeans (edamame)
- Split peas

Protein

Try to eat five or six servings of protein per day.

A proper portion of protein is the size of the palm of one hand.

The protein you eat should come from sources of lean meats, poultry, fish and eggs, dairy and some vegetable and grain sources.

- Lean meats (chicken, bison), poultry, fish
- Eggs
- Dairy
- Tofu, chia sees (Salba), quinoa and hemp seed (vegan option)
- Beans- bought dry and cooked yourself (vegan option)
- Nuts, Seeds and Nut Butters (vegan option)

Have a substantial amount of protein but a great deal of fat. While this fat is healthy, you don't want to eat too much of it. Serving: One scant handful of nuts or two tablespoons of nut butter per day.

Carbs from Fruits and Vegetables

A proper serving of fruits and veggies is four to six servings of fresh produce per day.

Serving size for fruits and veggies is two cupped hands.

Complex Carbs From Fruit

- Artichokes
- Apples
- Asparagus
- Berries
- Beet Greens
- Dried fruits in moderation
- Broccoli
- Grapefruit
- Brussels sprouts
- Grapes

- Cabbage
- Kiwi
- Cauliflower
- Lychee
- Celery
- Mango
- Cucumbers
- Melon
- Eggplant
- Oranges
- Kale
- Papaya
- Lettuce
- Passion Fruit
- Okra
- Pears
- Onions
- Plums
- Spinach
- Pomegranate
- Tomatoes
- Turnip Greens
- Watercress
- Zucchini

Healthy Fats

Your body needs unsaturated fats with high omega 3. They help keep your skin stay hydrated and lustrous, cells working properly, and aid in digestion and can also decrease inflammation. You need these fats to help you stay lean.

Serving: 15 percent of your diet should come from healthy fats from nuts, seeds, healthy oils and fish.

- Almonds
- Avocado oil
- Cashews
- Flax seed
- Hazelnut oil
- Olive oil
- Pecans
- Pumpkinseed oil
- Safflower oil
- Sunflower seeds
- Walnuts
- Coconut oil

Understanding The Role Of Fiber

So what is Dietary Fiber? Why is it important?

Dietary fiber comes from plant food like whole grain, fruits and vegetables. It is the part of plant food which resists digestion or absorption by the body. You may wonder if fiber resists digestion, basically does not add to the calorie intake, what is its function in the body? The fact is, a diet rich in fiber can do wonders - the benefits range from regular bowel movements, satiety, less chance of overeating, maintaining body weight, to lowering cholesterol levels and blood glucose response after a meal. Actually overwhelming scientific evidence has led to many health bodies around the world to approve health claims on fiber!

There are two types of fiber, one which is soluble and the other insoluble, and both are important. Both types can be found in a food, but some foods could be a better source of either one. Soluble fiber forms a gel in the body, which can delay the emptying of the stomach. It is also usually associated with its ability to lower cholesterol, and growth of friendly bacteria.

Insoluble fiber absorbs water and adds bulk which helps the wastes to pass more quickly though the body and key to preventing constipation.

Soluble fiber is found in barley, oats, nuts, rajma, channa, peas, apples, pears, flax seeds. Insoluble fiber is found in whole grain cereals - wheat bran/whole wheat flour, brown rice, nuts, seeds, dates and vegetables.

Most people want to live long and healthy lives. Because of this many are willing to change the way they eat and the things that they do in order to make this more likely. One of the changes that can be helpful is to include more dietary fiber in your diet. This is an important area where many people's diets are lacking and can easily be improved by sensible eating.

Dietary fiber has a number of significant benefits. First of all, it can help with weight loss since it makes you feel fuller as you eat the fibrous food and so you end up eating less. It also can help to lower cholesterol, and it might even help to prevent some types of cancer, such as colon cancer.

There are essentially two sorts of dietary fiber present in food and these are beneficial in different ways. The two types are soluble fiber and insoluble fiber. Plants contain both types of fiber in different quantities depending upon the plant.

If you want to eat foods rich in soluble fiber then you have to eat fruit, vegetables, lentils, beans and similar. If you want to eat insoluble fiber then consider such food as brown rice, whole meal bread. Also fruit and vegetables contain ample insoluble fiber as well as soluble fiber.

It is important to drink plenty of fluids such as water, tea, coffee or low calorie squash when eating fibrous foods to allow it to work properly. Food fiber soaks up water like a sponge. It swells as it absorbs water present in the stomach and thus can help to produce a feeling of being full.

Most foods that are high in fiber are low in fat. The exceptions are seeds and nuts. The average adult should consume about eighteen grams of fiber each day, although that figure is under review and may be increased to as much as thirty grams a day. In the United Kingdom, the average person consumes just twelve grams each day and this is far too little.

Dietary fiber helps to lower blood cholesterol. It also assists in keeping blood glucose and insulin levels stable, making it an important factor in reducing the risk of heart disease and type2 diabetes.

Sufferers of diverticulitis, hemorrhoids, and constipation can also find some relief of their symptoms and have fewer problems if they begin to eat a diet that is higher in fiber. Fiber really helps to regulate your system and keep you from getting constipated.

Dietary fiber is found in plant foods only. Canned and frozen produce still has just as much fiber as fresh. However, if you remove seeds or peel the produce you will lose some of the fiber that the food contains.

Since these foods are the cornerstone of a healthy diet anyway and have many other components of excellent nutrition value, such as vitamins and minerals and phytochemicals, it is a good idea to eat more of them, even if it weren't for the added benefits of the fiber they contain.

One obvious way of eating fiber is in the morning with your breakfast. If you start with a bowl of healthy cereal such as wheat biscuits, corn flakes or porridge you are well on the way to boosting your fiber intake.

However many of today's more popular breakfast cereals are devious in their presentation. They are very high in sugars and often much lower in fiber than is imagined. Check the label of your favorite 'sweet cereal' and compare it with that of a more basic version. You will be astonished by the figures. If you or your child wants to have a sweet or 'fruity' breakfast cereal, why not get the unsweetened variety and add your own chopped fruit. It is really tasty, but it also gives a double whammy of fiber while delivering a wholesome and healthy breakfast.

Although there are supplements available that you can use to increase your intake of dietary fiber, these are not recommended as much as getting your fiber from food. First of all you don't get the other added benefits of eating the food, but also they might not be as beneficial for other reasons.

These supplements might interfere with some drugs you might be taking, while food would not. There are also different types of fiber in foods, although it is still not clear which types provide which benefits, so you might be missing out on the benefits you desire if you take a supplement containing the wrong type of fiber.

Another reason for eating your fiber in vegetables and fruit rather than taking a supplement is that they enhance the look of any dish and thus encourage healthy and enjoyable eating.

Finally, remember the recommendations about eating five portions of fruit or vegetables a day? Well, now you understand why this advice is so sound. Dietary fiber keeps you healthy, reduces cholesterol and helps to keep the heart healthy. It can help you reduce weight and lessens the chance of developing diabetes.Dietary fiber is truly a magic ingredient in our food and one that it is good to know more about and, thus, appreciate the value of.

CHAPTER TWO

CLEAN EATING: FOODS TO AVOID

Eating clean food list and what to avoid

1. Stay away from things that were made in factories.

This includes all types of junk food and most types of processed food. Ice cream, sausages, ketchup, breakfast cereals, candy, pizza, low-fat dairy and many, many more. A decent rule of thumb is to evaluate if what you are going to eat looks similar to what it might have looked like in its natural state. If not, then you probably don't want to eat it. This rule has a few exceptions such as high-fat dairy, which is considered healthy for us because of its high vitamin K2 content.

2. Choose the less processed option.

It can be costly to always eat organic food, and is not compulsory doing that unless you have the money to afford it. There is however often a healthier, lesser processed option. For example, if grass-fed beef is too expensive for you, then buy grain-fed beef but a variety that looks natural and doesn't have a lot of additives in it.

3. Eat plants and animals.

When we were hunter-gatherers, back in the Paleolithic era, we ate plants and animals. It seems logical that these foods would keep us healthy, since our bodies were genetically designed for them. Optimal foraging theory works here, if the food you are about to eat has the possibility of being harvested in nature without taking many days in order to obtain a meal's worth of nutrition, then it is probably fine to eat.

4. Avoid modern disease promoting foods.

Sugar is our number one enemy here, followed closely by processed omega-6 vegetable oils and wheat. If you are able to cut these three foods out of your life completely, then you are already well on your way towards a healthy lifestyle. 80% of the health benefits of eating healthy are from cutting out these three foods.

If you follow this eating clean food list, and these tips on what to avoid, then It is guaranteed that your health will improve dramatically. The main causes of modern health problems are an unhealthy diet and lack of exercise.

Foods to avoid in The Clean eating Diet

- All packaged, canned, and processed foods and drinks, especially those that contain additives, preservatives, and other chemicals
- Sandwiches, hamburgers, pizza, wheat pasta, sushi, tomato-based sauces, tofu dishes, wheat-noodle dishes, anything with Asian soy sauces, baked potato, omelets and egg-based breakfast, wheat and corn tortillas, burritos, empanadas, lattes, cappuccinos, all coffee drinks, and desserts of all kinds unless they are fruit salad or plain fruit
- Dairy and eggs: all, including whey and butter substitutes; all butter and mayonnaise, including ghee
- Grains: white rice, wheat, corn, barley, spelt, kamut, rye, triticale, oats (even gluten-free)

- Fruits and vegetables: oranges, orange juice, grapefruit, bananas, strawberries, corn, creamed vegetables, nightshades (tomatoes, peppers, eggplant, and potatoes)
- Animal protein: pork (bacon), beef, veal, sausage, cold cuts, canned meats, frankfurters/hot dogs, shellfish, any raw meats and fish
- Vegetable protein: soybean products (soy sauce, soybean oil in processed foods, tempeh, tofu, soy milk, soy yogurt, textured vegetable protein). Note that miso and fermented soy sauce are listed as okay.
- Nuts and seeds: peanuts and peanut butter
- Oils: shortening, processed oils, canola oil, most salad dressings and spreads
- Drinks: alcohol, fruit juice (unless fresh-pressed), caffeinated beverages including coffee and black tea, soft drinks / soda including low-calorie sodas, "natural" sodas, or energy drinks
- Sweeteners: white and brown refined sugars, honey, maple syrup, high-fructose corn syrup HFCS, agave, evaporated cane juice
- Condiments: regular chocolate (with dairy and sugar), ketchup, relish, chutney, most jams and jellies (made with sugar), barbecue sauce, teriyaki sauce, gum, breath mints
- A few things to watch out for
- Corn starch is often present in baking powder, beverages, and processed foods
- Vinegar, mayonnaise, and some mustard can come from wheat or corn
- Breads advertised as gluten-free still might contain oats, spelt, kamut, or rye
- Many canned tunas contain textured vegetable protein TVP, which is from soy; look for low-salt versions, which tend to be pure tuna with no fillers

- Multi-grain rice cakes are not just rice. Be sure to purchase plain brown rice cakes
- "Natural flavors" can mean MSG
- Many amaranth and millet flake cereals contain oat or corn
- Try to avoid xanthium gum whenever possible. Guar gum is a better choice for fillers but not for those who are overly sensitive to gums
- In general, avoid/minimize acid-forming foods: alcohol, beans* (most kinds), beef, chicken, corn, dairy products, eggs, fish*, grains, lamb*, nuts*, pork, plums & prunes, rice, sodas, shellfish, sugar, sweet potatoes, tomatoes (processed), turkey, unripe fruit (note those marked * may be eaten according to the guidelines)
- Watch out for these common food and packaging sources of heavy-metal exposure:
- Aluminum – aluminum cooking vessels, baking powder, aluminum cans, milk and milk products, drinking water, pickled foods, color additives, vanilla powder, table salt, seasonings, bleached flour, American cheese
- Cadmium – drinking water, soft water from galvanized pipes, soft drinks, refined wheat flour, canned evaporated milk, processed foods, oysters
- Lead: drinking water from lead plumbing, vegetables from lead-contaminated soil, canned fruits and juices, canned evaporated milk, milk from animals fed in lead-contaminated land, organ meats, eating utensils
- Mercury: grain seeds treated with methyl mercury fungicide, predator fish, and certain lake fish
- Arsenic: insecticide residues on fruits and vegetables, drinking water, well water, seawater, wine

HEALTH BENEFITS OF FRUITS AND VEGETABLES

1. Nutrition and Antioxidants

The first reason that fruits and veggies are healthy lies in the fact that they contain high amounts of nutrition. These foods are packed with vitamins, minerals, and antioxidants, which means that they provide your body with the nutrition that it needs to be healthy and well. When you are eating a sufficient amount of nutrition, your major organs can function properly-which means that your body can fight off disease and illness, build, grow and repair.

2. Low in Calories

Fruits and vegetables are high in nutrition, but they are low in calories. Keeping a moderate calorie intake is a great way to manage weight and also prevent other conditions that correspond with high calorie consumption. Research studies have showed that moderate calorie consumption is linked with a healthier lifestyle.

3. Avoid Disease and Illness

Because fruits and veggies provide you will good nutrition and a healthy amount of fiber, your body is able to prevent serious illnesses and disease. Multiple sources have linked a high consumption of fresh produce with a lower risk of serious diseases such as heart disease, cancer, diabetes, and strokes.

4. Control Free Radicals

You have probably heard the term "free radicals" before, and you probably know that high levels of free radicals can be harmful to our health-they may even be the cause of cancer and early aging. Eating plenty of fruits and vegetables will help your body to get rid of these harmful free radicals, the antioxidants that are found in dark colored produce can effective reduce the free radicals in the body.

5. Fiber, Fiber, Fiber!

Eating plenty of fiber is essential for health and wellness, fiber helps to keep the digestive system running smoothly and it also helps the body to get rid of toxins and waste. Fruits and vegetables are a great source of healthy fiber; they will help you to avoid illness and disease by keeping your colon clean and healthy.

You definitely won't go wrong by consuming more fruits and veggies, make it a point to include these healthy foods in your meals every day. There are many options to choose from, be sure to eat a variety of whole foods in order to have optimal health.

CHAPTER THREE

HEALTHY HABITS FOR CLEAN EATING

Take an inventory of your pantry and refrigerator. Great now let's do a Spring Cleaning and talk about the rules of clean eating. This isn't about another diet or even depriving yourself. It is a lifestyle change in learning to eat healthy and clean. It involves planning healthy meals for the week, but first you must develop healthy habits.

Habit #1: Eat six meals per day, one every three hours. This sounds unbelievable and it is the opposite of what most popular diets tell you, but eating better foods more frequently actually increases your metabolism and keeps your energy levels high all day. Eating small meals throughout the day will also stabilize blood sugar levels and cravings will stop. When you eat just three meals a day or less, your sugar levels dip and you are more likely to eat unhealthy snacks.

Metabolism can be compared to a wood burning fire. As long as you keep putting wood on that fire, the fire is going to do what? That's right keep burning. If you quit putting wood on that fire, what is going to happen? That's right it is going to go out. This is just like metabolism. If you try to starve to lose weight, your metabolism is going to come to a screeching halt or slow weigh down. Then when you do eat, your body is going to store and hold on to every ounce for dear life. So it is best to feed your metabolism every 3 hours or so to keep it going.

Habit #2: Never skip meals, especially breakfast. How many of you skip breakfast? The research shows that people who skip breakfast, they gain more weight. You think you are saving on calories, but skipping breakfast will lead you to snack before lunch or overeat at lunch because you are hungry.

Habit #3: Don't eat calorie dense foods that offer no nutritional value. Processed and fast foods such as French fries, chips, donuts, cookies and candy are a nutritional wasteland. The calories in these foods are considered "empty" because they give you a quick burst of energy but no vitamins, nutrients or natural ingredients. You usually have a sugar high followed by a crash that leaves you without energy and feeling hungry soon after. These foods tend to generate cravings for even more energy calories because you never really feel satisfied.

Habit #4: Think about portion sizes, not calorie counting. It is important to keep in mind how much fuel your body really needs. Most portion sizes in restaurants like Applebees, and Chilis are nearly twice the size of a true serving. You could order salads and appetizers, but you have to be careful of which appetizer you order! Fried cheese curds are yummy; however, they are fried and contain a lot of fat. At home, it is easy to clear your plate or eat that last little bit in the pan to avoid leftovers which is in effect overeating. And, it is never just a little bit!!! So, here are some guidelines... a serving of protein should fit in the palm of your hand or roughly the size of a deck of cards. A serving of complex carbohydrates from grains should fit in the cup of your hand. While a serving of complex carbs from veggies should fit in the palm of two open hands. Fruits should fit in one open hand.

Habit #5: Drink a minimum of 8 glasses of water a day. Staying hydrated is essential for good health as 80% of our body is water. When you are low, you will show symptoms such as fatigue, irritability, headaches and constipation. Now, if you are one of those people who think water is boring and you don't like the taste, you can flavor your water. Cut up some lemon, limes or oranges and put them in your water bottle. It doesn't take a lot to infuse flavor and antioxidants. If strawberries are on sale, you can add these to your water. Just make sure you take out the strawberries within 48 hours as they are not acidic and can grow bacteria.

Habit #6: Eliminate sweets from your diet especially white sugar. Candies, cakes, cookies and ice cream are obvious. However, sugar has a way of sneaking in the most seemingly healthy snacks and is often the reason you can't lose those last pesky 5-10 pounds. Examples include sweetened yogurts, processed peanut butter, granola, protein bars and canned fruits in syrup. Many condiments and salad dressings contain sugar or high fructose corn syrup that stops your progress in its tracks without the sweet taste!

Habit #7: Eat fruits and veggies. Clean eating does not have to be boring. Processed foods seem healthier because of all the unhealthy ingredients and fats. Your taste buds will recalibrate by the intense flavor of food without artificial ingredients. Some of my favorite nonfat condiments that heighten taste include fresh and dried herbs, horseradish, garlic, mustards, ginger, vinegars, Worcestershire sauce, citrus fruit, freshly made salsas, pureed fruit and veggie based sauces, unsweetened apple butter or sauce, Bragg's, and low sodium tamari or soy sauce

What Are Healthy Good Eating Habits?

We all need good eating habits. We all need a healthy life. It is in our interest to stay fit and healthy, which means being full of energy, we need to sleep well at night, have peace of mind and be disease free. All this will give a sense of well-being. So what is a healthy well-balanced diet?

There are two elements of a well-balanced diet; these are eating the correct amount of food for how active you are, and eating a range of foods.

In order to achieve all or some of the above, we have to practice healthy lifestyle with good food and exercise. To be sluggish is not being healthy. To be healthy we must be both mentally and physically fit.

Good eating habits by eating healthy food can keep you strong and healthy. As the main reason for disease and ill-health is bad food habits, try to avoid processed and refined food.

A simple change of diet can improve your health within a short period. The choice of foods in your diet ought to consist of a sufficient amount of fruit and vegetables, whole grain varieties of bread, rice, potatoes, pasta and other starchy foods.

Some meat, eggs, beans, fish and non-dairy sources of protein also some milk and dairy foods. Also keep foods high in fats and sugars to a minimum.

Eating well plays an important part in continuing good health. Here are some tips covering some of the basic that can help make the difference with good eating habits.

• Have your breakfast as it gives you energy to face the day.

• Drink between 6-8 glasses of water a day.

• Do not eat more than 6 grams of salt a day if you are an adult. Use sea salt or cook without salt if you can.

• Eat at least two portions of fish a week including an oily fish such as sardines or mackerel.

• Have fruit and vegetables at least five portions a day.

• You need energy so include starchy foods.

• Cut down on sugar and saturated fat.

• Do not overwork the digestive system eat small meals regularly.

• Have a piece of fruit as a healthy snack between meals to control your energy level.

• Do not get too hungry that you overeat at mealtimes

• Eat slowly - enjoy your food.

• Try to eat one well balance meal with the family to promote good eating habits to the others.

• Avoid white bread, white rice, pastries, sodas and high processes foods.

• Drinking moderately has health benefits although this is not recommended to everyone.

• A daily multivitamin with vitamin D has health benefits.

Developing good eating habits mean you will meet your daily requirements of vitamins, minerals and other nutrients. It also reduces the risk of obesity, high blood pressure, heart disease, type 2 diabetes and certain forms of cancer.

To improve and maintain good general health, healthy eating is vital to lowering health risks such as obesity; provide water and essential nutrients to the body. The healthy body gives energy when needed, and do not have excessive weight due to too much and inadequate consumption of food.

Five Healthy Eating Habits To Develop This Week

Let's face it, it's not an easy thing to improve your daily eating habits on a consistent basis. This is especially true if you have been eating in an unhealthy matter for quite some time and are desperately trying to turn this around. Naturally it's going to be tough to change your habits and kick the fast food habit if you're used to eating that daily. Nevertheless, if you have a goal to lose weight, one of the first things you must get a strong handle on is your daily nutrition. Weight loss success is 70% dependent on your nutrition so it's vital you get a good handle on this first.

Therefore here are five ways you can develop healthy eating habits this week and leapfrog right to the forefront of a healthy lifestyle.

Make a list of two healthy meals you want to prepare this week.

If you want to eat in a more healthy manner that means you have to be willing to ditch the fast food and pizza delivery (at least for a bit) and start using your own kitchen to prepare meals. It may sound a bit foreign to you especially if you are not used to cooking in your kitchen, nevertheless this could be the number one healthy habit that will get you to accomplish your weight loss goal. Let's keep it simple when starting out and just write down a list of one or two meals (ingredients) that you would like to prepare this upcoming week.

Take a moment to search the Internet for healthy meals that look appealing to you. As you make your shopping list, double-check you have written everything you'll need to prepare the meal(s) and you'll soon have wonderful healthier meals right at home and won't have to rely on that fattening fast food.

Immediately portion the food into containers.

One of the best reasons for preparing food at home, aside from enjoying a well-portioned meal, is that you'll be able to create 3-5 meals from that one cooking episode. If you double or even triple the amount of ingredients, you will guarantee there will be plenty leftover to pack/freeze for future meals or immediately portion the extra into plastic travel containers so you'll have fantastic lunches to go. If you don't have a decent supply of travel containers, add them to your shopping list since these will become invaluable tools for your healthy eating efforts.

Be mindful of the drinks you consume.

Drinks can be sneaky daggers in the weight loss process since most people don't consider liquids as potential dangers. However when you look carefully at the nutritional content of soda, juice, energy drinks, and specialty coffees, you may be surprised at how high the calorie count is not to mention the sugar content you'll find in each serving. Since you're focusing on healthy eating habits, do away with these types of beverages and try to only drink water, black coffee, or other near-0 calorie option like tea. You'll be pleasantly delighted at how many calories you'll do away with especially if you were a heavy soda or juice drinker.

Use smaller plates and drink water with each meal.

This may sound like an unusual tip but using smaller plates really does help control the portion size consumed at meals. Eating too much food at meals is usually what packs on the excess weight. Our bodies simply do not need that much food to function efficiently. Problem is, you need to get used to eating less at meals, but that is where the water really comes into play and helps out. The portion on a small-sized plate will look like a lot of food and when you tie that in with a large glass of water, you will get full on much less than you may have been used to in the past.

Travel snacks and lunches for work.

This last healthy eating tip links right back to the first. When you cook food at home, plan to make extra to ensure you have leftovers. This leftover food can now become travel meals for work and when you toss in a couple healthy snacks to compliment your lunch, the entire time you're away from home will be nutritious and conducive to weight loss. Just don't slip on your choice of beverages when you're away from home. If it's possible, keep a pack of water bottles at work somewhere so you'll always have them handy and won't need to visit the vending machine any longer.

When you think about it, you can get a 36 pack of water bottles for around $4, whereas how much would 36 sodas from the vending machine cost over time? Not only will you be saving a lot of money, but you'll also save your body from having to ingest 5,400 calories.

HOW TO EAT CLEAN

1. Shop the outer ring of the grocery store. The outer ring of the grocery store contains foods including fruits, vegetables, and unprocessed meats. It will include dairy products that range from lightly processed to highly processed. When you go towards the center of the store you will find more foods that are heavily processed which may contain a long list of ingredients.

2. Read food labels. We talk about "processed" food as if it is the enemy. But we also need to define what that means. Processing can be as simple as turning a product that isn't in an edible state to a form that we will consume in our diet. To the extreme, processing can be adding colors, fillers, additives and chemicals to alter the taste, color and texture of a food to be more appealing to the consumer. Reading the label will help you understand where the difference lies. Look at the ingredient list and ask yourself the following questions.

• Are there more than 5 ingredients?

• Do I understand what each ingredient is?

(Sometimes added vitamins or minerals may be words you don't understand. Check out the products you buy and do some research to find out the definition of words you don't know, and then consider if you want to buy that product in the future).

• Does it have added sugars and where is that on the list of ingredients?

(The higher in the list, the greater the quantity of that ingredient)?

• Does it have added fats and what is the source of that fat - is it a source that I choose to include in my diet to nourish myself well?

• Does it contain additives, fillers or food dyes?

• Does it contain ingredients that you suspect you may be sensitive too?

3. Prepare your own food. In our culture with busy lives today buying prepared foods can be appealing to simplify your life. Unfortunately, with that your diet may not be as clean as you would like. Make a plan for three - five meals that you can prepare for dinner each week.

BENEFITS OF CLEAN EATING

Clean eating is one of the best things you can do for your health and wellbeing. It's simple, eat better and you'll look and feel better. Our cleanse guide is packed full of tips to help you start, download it here.

So many people confuse eating well with putting on weight. It's a big misconception since you need to eat to stop your body from storing food as fat, 3 good meals a day and 2 snacks will get that metabolism fired up! And don't forget to throw in some chillies/turmeric and cayenne pepper!

Following a clean diet is extremely important and getting in the right mix of nutrients can help prevent some of the less desired symptoms of ageing.

So if you haven't yet, here's why you need to start clean eating.

1. More energy

A balanced diet full of complex carbs while reducing sugar intake will give you more sustained energy throughout the day.

Combining complex carbs with protein gives you an energy boost without the inevitable crash that sugar gives.

2. Detoxifies Your Body

Clean eating rids the body of toxins, something we naturally become way less efficient at as we age. Detoxifying your body means your liver and stomach will be able to work more effectively, you'll have better circulation, improved skin, a stronger immune system and clearer cognitive function.

3. Aids With Weight Loss

Although eating at a deficit will always result in weight loss no matter what you eat, a clean diet full of fibrous foods and an adequate amount of protein will satiate you much more than junk and processed foods. This will also help your body composition improve by losing fat and retaining lean mass.

4. Eat Your Greens!

Believe it or not, it's possible to take years off your appearance by eating the right foods. You can even reverse some parts of ageing if you increase your intake of certain super foods. Following a diet rich in antioxidants, omega 3 oils, anti-inflammatories (we love turmeric!) and amino acids contribute to a glowing and plumper complexion.

5. Balances Hormones

Fat is one of the most important macronutrients for balanced hormones and increasing your intake of healthy fats through avocado, nut butter and eggs will stabilize hormone levels.

See our free clean eating plan for more, where we have recipe ideas, meal plans and everything you'll need to clean up your diet! And don't forget to DRINK plenty of water, this will keep you full and hydrated.

PROS AND CONS OF A CLEAN EATING DIET

As with any diet, it is important to understand the pros and cons of clean eating before deciding to adopt it as a lifestyle or diet. Make sure to look at each side carefully to make sure it fits your goals and lifestyle.

Pros of a Clean Eating Diet

Focused on whole and natural foods including mostly vegetables, fruits, unprocessed whole grains, and lean proteins

Leads to weight loss for many

Shown to have many health benefits including increased energy, cardiovascular benefits, digestive benefits, and more

Can be used as a general eating philosophy or as part of a healthy diet with calorie limits

Provides many nutrients when the person eats a well-balanced diet

Cons of a Clean Eating Diet

Can be hard to follow for some people because you must eliminate certain foods including sugar and processed foods

Can be expensive as you increase your intake of vegetables, fruits, lean proteins, nuts, and organic foods if you choose organic

Without a calorie limit, some people may overeat and gain weight even when eating clean

Participants need to monitor their meals to make sure they are eating a well-balanced diet to get needed nutrients

Involves more food preparation and cooking than some other diets since most foods begin in a whole and natural state

CHAPTER FOUR

CLEAN EATING BREAKFAST RECIPES

CLEAN EATING ONE EGG OMELET

INGREDIENTS

1 whole egg

⅛ tsp. onion powder

⅛ tsp. dried thyme

1-2 tsp. butter or oil

1 slice cheese

INSTRUCTIONS

In a small bowl, use a fork to whisk together the egg, onion powder and dried thyme.

Warm the oil in a small pan and pour the whisked egg into the pan, ensuring it reaches all the edges. If you end up with some raw egg on top, simply tip the pan a bit while lifting the edge or your omelet so that the raw egg can run underneath at the edge.

Flip the omelet and add cheese. Let it cook for just just long enough to warm the cheese, fold in half and transfer to your plate.

CLEAN EATING FAMILY FRITTATA

INGREDIENTS

8 large eggs

¼ cup parmesan cheese

1 tbsp. garlic powder

1 tbsp. coconut oil or oil of preference

5 stalks asparagus, sliced thin

¼ large, yellow onion, chopped fine

4 small shiitake mushrooms

Enough hand grated cheddar to cover the top of the frittata

INSTRUCTIONS

Preheat oven to 350 F.

Crack your eggs into a medium mixing bowl and whisk for 1-2 minutes to get the eggs well combined.

Whisk the parmesan and garlic powder into the eggs.

Warm the oil in a large skillet and saute the asparagus, onions and mushroom

When they are mostly cooked, turn off the heat and pour the eggs into the pan. Top with a layer of shredded cheese.

Place pan in the oven and bake for approximately 30 minutes or until a knife pulls out clean when inserted into the center.

Slice like a pizza and serve! For regular clean eaters, serve with a slice of whole grain bread or a side of fruit.

CLEAN EATING BREAKFAST BURGERS

INGREDIENTS:

4 egg whites

2 teaspoons olive oil

1 tablespoon salsa (clean, of course)

1/4 avocado

1 whole grain burger bun

DIRECTIONS:

Scramble the eggs in the olive oil in a medium-sized pan. Stir in the salsa and immediately remove pan from heat.

Assemble your burger using the eggs, avocado and the bun.

BLUEBERRY CRUMB CAKE MUFFINS

Ingredients:

1/2 cup unsweetened applesauce

1 small banana, peeled

2 eggs

1 egg white

1 cup unsweetened almond milk

1 TBSP pure vanilla extract

1 TBSP pure maple syrup

1 cup gluten-free oat flour

1 cup coconut flour

1/2 cup Stevia in the Raw

2 tsp baking powder

1/4 tsp sea salt

1 1/2 cups frozen blueberries

Directions:

1. Heat oven to 375 degrees Fahrenheit.

2. Using a large food processor or blender, puree applesauce and banana until smooth.

3. Add eggs and process for approximately 45 seconds.

4. Add remaining wet ingredients and mix.

5. Add dry ingredients and mix thoroughly.

6. Remove blade from food processor and fold blueberries into batter mixture.

7. Add to muffin tin and bake for 17-20 minutes until golden brown.

BANANA PROTEIN PANCAKES

In a blender mix:

1 banana

1 whole egg

1 egg white

1 scoop plant based vanilla protein powder

Dash of cinnamon

Pinch of baking soda

Pinch of baking powder

Blend until smooth.

In a bowl stir banana mixture with small pieces of strawberry. Cook medium sized pancakes in skillet over med-low heat. You also could use blueberries instead of strawberries. They're sweet enough to not need any syrup or honey. Serve with scrambled egg whites, steamed spinach and Ezekiel toast.

GLUTEN FREE BLUEBERRY BURST OATMEAL BAKE

Ingredients:

1 cup Gluten Free Rolled Oats

1 cup Gluten Free Quick Cooking Oats

1/4 cup Gluten Free Oat Flour (optional)

1/4 cup Stevia in the Raw

1/2 tsp Baking Powder

1/4 tsp Salt

2 Tbsp Pure Maple Syrup or Honey (optional)

1/2 tsp Pure Vanilla Extract (avoid HFCS)

2 Egg Whites

1/2 cup Unsweetened Almond Milk

1 cup Organic Blueberries

Directions:

1. Preheat oven to 350 degrees

2. Spray 8" pan with non stick spray

3. Combine all ingredients, except blueberries, and mix thoroughly

4. Once ingredients are combined, fold in blueberries

5. Bake for 20 minutes or until lightly browned on top

HEALTHY CAKE BATTER PANCAKES

Ingredients:

1/3 cup gluten free oat flour

3 Tbsp liquid egg whites

3 Tbsp unsweetened almond milk

1/2 tsp - 1 tsp pure vanilla extract (avoid HFCS)

1 tspNatvia sweetener (or sweetener of your choice)

Less than 1/4 tsp baking powder

Less than 1/4 tsp baking soda

Less than 1/4 tsp salt

Directions:

Add all ingredients to a mixing bowl & stir to combine. The batter will seem thick but keep stirring.

Coat (or spray) pan with olive oil or coconut oil to prevent sticking.

Add batter once pan is warm.

Cook for approx 2 minutes on each side or until slightly browned.

CHOCOLATE ALMOND OATMEAL PROTEIN SHAKE

Ingredients:

1 c unsweetened vanilla almond milk

1 banana, frozen and peeled

2 TBSP natural, unsalted almond butter

1 scoop Chocolate Protein Powder

1/4 cup Bob's Red Mill Gluten-Free Quick Cooking Oats

1/3 cup ice

Directions: Blend in a blender or food processor until desired consistency is achieved.

CHOCOLATE PEANUT BUTTER PROTEIN SHAKE

Ingredients:

2 oz liquid egg whites (pasteurized)

4-6 oz unsweetened vanilla almond milk

1 packet/scoop TLS chocolate whey protein powder

1 Tbsp natural peanut butter or almond butter

1 Tbsp cocoa powder

Stevia, to taste

A few ice cubes

Directions:

Blend all ingredients together & enjoy

OVERNIGHT OATS WITH CHOCOLATE AND STRAWBERRY

INGREDIENTS

OATS

¾ cup old-fashioned oats

1 tablespoon granulated sugar

1 tablespoon cocoa powder

½ to ¾ cup milk (such as whole, skim, almond, soy or coconut)

TOPPINGS

1 cup yogurt

½ cup sliced strawberries

DIRECTIONS

1. In a 1-pint mason jar, mix the oats with the sugar and cocoa powder to combine.

2. Add the milk to the jar with the oats. (If you prefer thicker oatmeal, use less milk.)

3. Screw on the lid and refrigerate overnight, about 8 hours.

4. In the morning, top the oatmeal with yogurt and sliced strawberries. Eat immediately or screw the top on and take it on the go.

MINT CACAO NIB PROTEIN GREEN SMOOTHIE

INGREDIENTS

2 frozen bananas, diced

1 cup packed organic spinach leaves

1 cup unsweetened almond milk

2 scoops protein powder of choice

10 mint leaves OR 1/4 teaspoon mint or peppermint extract

2 tablespoons Cacao nibs (or vegan chocolate chips)

INSTRUCTIONS

Place all ingredients besides cocoa nibs in a blender and blend on high until ingredients are smooth and well combined. Next, add cacao nibs to the blender and pulse a few times until they slightly break up in the smoothie. Serve immediately.

KALE QUICHE WITH A CHEDDAR-RICE CRUST

INGREDIENTS

CRUST

2 cups cooked rice

2 egg whites

½ cup shredded cheddar cheese

QUICHE

5 large eggs

1 cup milk

Salt and freshly ground black pepper

3 green onions, thinly sliced

½ bunch kale, roughly torn

DIRECTIONS

1. Preheat the oven to 375°F. Lightly grease a 9-inch pie plate.

2. MAKE THE CRUST: In a large bowl, mix the rice with the egg whites and shredded cheese until well combined.

3. Using damp hands, press the rice mixture evenly into the pie plate. Bake until the crust begins to brown, 13 to 15 minutes. Cool slightly.

4. MAKE THE QUICHE: In a medium bowl, whisk the eggs with the milk to combine; season with salt and pepper to taste. Arrange the green onions and kale in an even layer in the prepared crust and then pour the egg mixture over it. (Note: Any exposed kale sticking out from the top of the egg custard will get crispy like kale chips.)

5. Bake until the egg mixture is set in the center, 25 to 30 minutes. Cool slightly before slicing and serving.

BAKED EGGS WITH RICOTTA AND KALE

Ingredients

10 oz. chopped kale

2 tsp. chopped garlic

¼ cup (28 g.) lite ricotta

¼ cup (28 g.) crumbled feta

½ tsp. dried lemon peel

4 large eggs

¼ cup (about 6) grape tomatoes (chopped or sliced)

Kosher Salt and fresh ground Pepper (to taste)

Cooking spray

Directions

Preheat your oven to 350°F. Place two small oven safe bowls on the oven as it heats.

Coat a large skillet with cooking spray.

Add the kale and sauté over medium high until wilted down and soft.

Add garlic and a little salt and pepper to taste (about ¼ tsp each).

In a small mixing bowl stir to combine the ricotta, feta, lemon peel, and a pinch of salt and pepper (about 1/8 tsp. each).

When oven is hot remove bowls and place them on a cookie sheet.

Divide the kale in half and fill each bowl with the kale.

Make two wells in each bowl of kale and crack an egg into each well (2 eggs per bowl).

Divide the cheese mixture in half and dot each kale-egg bowl with the cheese.

Bake the eggs for 20 to 25 minutes (until eggs are cooked to your liking and cheese has started to brown).

Top the bowls with the tomatoes and eat

BLUEBERRY FARRO YOGURT

INGREDIENTS

1cup farro

2cups water

1 1/2 cups frozen wild blueberries

1tablespoon honey

1tablespoon chia seeds

1tablespoon lemon zest (Meyer lemons are great for this!)

2containers Siggi's blueberry yogurt

INSTRUCTIONS

Place the farro and water in a small sauce pot, bring to a boil then reduce to a low simmer and cover. Cook until all the water is absorbed by the farro, about 20 minutes.

Meanwhile, make the blueberry jam by adding the blueberries and honey to another small sauce pot over medium heat. Cook for about 5 minutes until blueberries give off their liquid.

Add the chia seeds and lemon zest, reduce the heat to medium-low and continue cooking for about 10 more minutes, stirring frequently to help mash up the jam. When most of the liquid is gone and the jam has thickened, remove from heat.

Serve the yogurt, farro and blueberry jam together in a bowl.

ALMOND MANGO OVERNIGHT OATS

Ingredients

1/4 cup uncooked organic rolled oats

1/3 cup almond or soy milk

1/4 cup low-fat Greek yogurt

1-1/2 teaspoons dried chia seeds

1/8 teaspoon almond extract

1 teaspoon agave nectar or honey

1/4 cup diced mango (about half a sliced mango)

Directions

In a medium sized, resealable container combine dried oats, milk, yogurt, chia seeds, almond extract and agave nectar. Seal with the lid and shake until well incorporated.

Add mango and stir until well mixed. Reseal with the lid and refrigerate overnight, up to 2 days. Enjoy cold!

BREAKFAST QUICHE

Ingredients

8 large egg whites

1 whole egg

1 cup fresh baby spinach, torn or chopped

1/2 cup chopped veggies

1/4 cup feta cheese, fat-free

1/2 teaspoon black pepper

sea salt to taste

Directions

Preheat oven to 350 degrees. In a medium or large bowl mix all ingredients together until fully incorporated

Lightly spray fat-free cooking spray in muffin tin or 9" round cake pan and pour in mixture. If using muffin tin bake for approximately 22 minutes or until tops start to brown. If using round cake pan, bake for approximately

30 minutes or until top starts to brown. Allow 5 minutes to cool and enjoy!

BLUEBERRY BANANA PANCAKE

Ingredients

1 cup oat flour

1 cup white whole-wheat flour

2 1/4 teaspoons baking powder

1/2 teaspoon baking soda

1/4 teaspoon sea salt

2 eggs, slightly beaten

1/4 cup canola oil

1 banana, mashed

2 tablespoons agave nectar

1 cup almond milk

1/2 cup low-fat milk

1/2 cup fresh blueberries

Directions

In a large mixing bowl, whisk all dry ingredients together until fully incorporated. In a separate mixing bowl combine the rest of the ingredients, except blueberries. Combine wet mixture with the dry mixture and stir well.

Fold in blueberries. Heat skillet enough to sizzle a drip of water. Lightly spray fat-free cooking spray on skillet and pour on 1/4 cup of pancake mix.

Gently flip pancakes when center begins to bubble and the bottom is golden brown.

Enjoy with additional blueberries and banana and drizzle with agave nectar or 100% pure maple syrup.

QUINOA BERRY BOWL

Ingredients

1 cup quinoa

2 cups water

1 tablespoon vanilla

2 cups fresh blueberries

1 tablespoon of pure virgin coconut oil

1/2 teaspoon of powder cinnamon

Sea salt to add some taste

Directions

Preheat oven to 400 degrees. In a medium sauce pan, mix quinoa, water, vanilla and a pinch of salt. Bring water to a boil, cover and reduce to heat to a simmer for 15 minutes.

At this point, the liquid should be absorbed. In a separate bowl mix blueberries, melted coconut oil and cinnamon.

Spread this mixture on a parchment paper lined baking sheet and roast in the oven for 15 minutes or until soft and bubbly.

Serve quinoa topped with the roasted blueberry mix and top with fresh blueberries and slivered

OATMEAL POWER BOWL

Ingredients

1 ripe banana, mashed

2 tablespoons chia seeds

Heaping 1/3 cup organic rolled oats

1/4 teaspoon cinnamon

2/3 cup almond milk

1/3 cup water

Optional toppings: slivered almonds, sunflower seeds, cinnamon, dried cranberries. toasted coconut, nut butter, cinnamon, all spice

Directions

In a medium bowl, mash banana until smooth. Stir in chia seeds, milk, oats, cinnamon and water until fully incorporated. Cover and refrigerate overnight.

In the morning scoop oatmeal mixture into a medium pan and heat to a simmer then reduce heat immediately to medium-low stirring occasionally until heated throughout and mixture has thickened.

Pour oatmeal into a bowl and top with your favorite toppings

MUG APPLE MUFFIN

Ingredients

1 TBS coconut oil

2 TBS unsweetened apple sauce

1 egg

1/4 tsp vanilla

1 tsp agave nectar

2 TBS almond flour

1/2 tsp cinnamon

1/8 tsp baking powder

Pinch of salt

Streusel topping

1 tbs apple, finely chopped

Pinch of crumbled walnuts

Pinch of cold coconut oil

Directions

For Muffin – Melt coconut oil in microwave safe mug. Whisk in applesauce, egg, vanilla and agave nectar until completely incorporated. Add cinnamon, almond flour, baking powder and salt. Stir well. Microwave for 1 minute and 10 seconds.

For Streusel Topping – In a small dish combine apple, walnuts and coconut oil using a small rubber spatula and top muffin after microwaving.

CHAPTER FIVE

CLEAN EATING LUNCH RECIPES

SKINNY BROCCOLI & CHEESE TWICE BAKED POTATOES

Ingredients

3 Large golden sweet potatoes

2 cups Broccoli florets (fresh or frozen)

1/2 cup Plain nonfat Greek yogurt

2 tbsUnsweetened almond milk (or milk of choice)

4 slices Center cut bacon, cooked and crumbled

1/2 cup Cheddar cheese, shredded

1/4 cup Parmesan cheese, grated

1 tspGarlic powder

1/4 tspSalt

1/4 tspPepper

Topping

1/2 cup Cheddar cheese, shredded

Directions

- Bake the Potatoes: Scrub the potatoes, and prick several time with a fork or knife. Place on a baking sheet pan or plate (depending on cooking method you choose).
- Microwave: Cook potatoes on full power in the microwave for 5 minutes. Turn over, and continue to

cook for 2-5 minutes. When you can pierce potato easily with a fork. Remove from microwave and let cool until it you are able to handle potatoes.

- Oven: Roast potatoes at 425 degrees for 45-60 minutes or until you can pierce easily with a fork. Remove from oven and let cool until you are able to handle potatoes.

- Prepare the Filling: Preheat oven to 425 degrees (unless it is already preheated from baking potatoes) . Line a baking sheet pan with foil and spray with nonstick cooking spray.

- After potatoes have cooled, cut potatoes in half lengthwise. Use a spoon to scoop out flesh, saving 1 cup of the flesh of the potato for the filling in a medium bowl, (save the rest of the flesh for mashed potatoes or whatever you'd like!) Also, be sure you leave the sides thick enough so that the skin doesn't cave when stuffed.

- Steam broccoli until it is tender (you can do this in the microwave or in a pot of boiling water), or you are using frozen broccoli in steamer bag, cook for about 3-4 minutes in the microwave. Chop the steamed broccoli florets until they are very fine.

- Add broccoli to the medium bowl with the potato flesh. Add the rest of the ingredients, (except for the toppings). Scoop the filling back into the potato skins and place on baking pan.

- Bake for 15-20 minutes, or until cheese is melted to your liking. Let cool for about 5 minutes and top with Greek yogurt, additional bacon, chives, or toppings of choice if desired.

HONEY BACON WRAPPED CHICKEN TENDERS

Ingredients

1.25 lbsChicken tenders

12 slices Center cut bacon

1/3 cup Honey

1 tbsChili powder (or spice of choice)

Method

Preheat oven to 400 degrees. Line a rimmed baking sheet pan with foil and spray with cooking spray.

In a shallow dish, combine honey and chili powder.

Wrap each chicken tender with one slice of bacon and place on baking sheet pan. Coat bacon wrapped chicken tenders with the honey/chili mixture.

Bake for 20 to 25 minutes, until bacon is crisp and chicken is cooked through.

MEDITERRANEAN CRAB SALAD

INGREDIENTS

4 ounces mixed greens

6 cherry tomatoes cut in half

1/4 cup diced cucumber

1/4 cup diced Kalamata olives

2 ounces fresh crab

1 tablespoon extra virgin olive oil

1 tablespoon champagne vinegar

1 tablespoon fresh mint

fresh ground pepper to taste

1 ounce crumbled feta cheese (optional, omit if vegan)

INSTRUCTIONS

Combine first 6 ingredients together in a bowl.

Drizzle oil and vinegar over all ingredients.

Sprinkle with mint.

EDAMAME TOSSED ZOODLES WITH HONEY WALNUT VINAIGRETTE

INGREDIENTS

Dressing

1 tablespoon organic, raw honey

1 tablespoon of freshly squeezed orange juice

2 tablespoons sherry vinegar

1/4 fresh mint, diced

3 tablespoon walnut oil

Salad

2 large zucchinis

8 ounces of shelled edamame (frozen is easiest)

3 ounces of walnuts, coarsely chopped

INSTRUCTIONS

Place the honey in a glass bowl and microwave for 5-10 seconds so it's in liquid form. Whisk in the orange, sherry vinegar and mint. Then slowly add the oil, stirring until combined. Set the dressing aside.

Spiralize the zucchinis (instructions here). Place the zucchini strands over a colander, salt and allow to stand for 30 minutes so the moisture can release.

Bring a medium pot of salted water to a boil. Add the edamame and cook uncovered about 5 minutes until tender, but not soft. Drain and rinse with cold water.

Squeeze any remaining moisture from the zucchini and pat dry. Place zoodles in a glass bowl. Add the edamame and slowly incorporate the dressing (you may not need all of it for the one salad). Toss and top with walnuts.

CRAB SALAD LETTUCE CUPS {MAYONNAISE FREE}

INGREDIENTS

8 ounces fresh lump crab meat, picked with shells removed

1/4 teaspoon Old Bay (or to taste)

1 garlic clove, minced

1 tablespoon fresh basil, chopped

1 teaspoon Dijon mustard

1 teaspoon champagne vinegar

2 tablespoons extra virgin olive oil

1/4 cup cucumber, diced

1 avocado, cored and cut

About 8 baby romaine leaves

Instructions

Place crab in bowl and season with Old Bay.

In a medium bowl, place garlic, basil, Dijon and vinegar and whisk. Gradually add olive oil, stirring until combined.

Combine crab with vinaigrette and mix well. Fold in the cucumber and avocado.

Lay out the lettuce leaves and scoop the mixture down the middle, garnishing with a shake of Old Bay.

BAKED CHICKEN WITH PEPPERS & MUSHROOMS

INGREDIENTS

3 lbs chicken breasts or thighs, boneless & skinless

1 large garlic clove, grated

1/2 tsphimalayan pink salt

Ground black pepper, to taste

1 medium onion, finely chopped

10 brown mushrooms or 2 portobellos, chopped

2 large bell peppers, chopped

1 tbsp coconut or avocado oil

1 cup hard cheese like mozzarella or marble, shredded

Directions

Preheat oven to 425 degrees. Rinse chicken and if using breasts cut in half lengthwise. In a large baking dish, add chicken, garlic, salt and pepper. Mix well to coat evenly and spread in a single layer. Cover and bake for 20-25 minutes. Chicken is cooked when pale and surrounded by clear juices.

In the meanwhile, preheat large ceramic non-stick skillet on low-medium heat and swirl oil to coat. Add onion and saute for a few minutes, stirring occasionally. Add mushrooms and saute for a few more minutes, stirring occasionally. Add bell peppers and saute for 5 more minutes, stirring.

Remove chicken from the oven and turn broiler on High. Separate chicken a bit from each other and top each piece with vegetables (sprinkle around too) and top with cheese. Broil for 5 minutes or until cheese is melted. Serve hot with rice, quinoa or veggies.

Storage Instructions: Refrigerate in an airtight container for up to 3 days.

THAI TURKEY MEATBALLS IN 30 MINUTES

INGREDIENTS

For Meatballs:

2 lbs ground turkey, extra lean

1 cup zucchini, shredded & liquid squeezed out

1 tbsp fish sauce

1/4 cup green onions, finely chopped

2 tbsp basil, finely chopped

2 tsp ginger, grated

2 garlic cloves, grated

1 tsp red curry paste

2 tbsp coconut milk, light (canned)

1/8 tsp red pepper flakes

Cooking spray

For the Sauce:

1 + 1/2 cup coconut milk, light (canned)

3 tbsp tomato paste

1 tsp red curry paste

1 tsp fish sauce

1/8 tsp red pepper flakes, more to taste

5-6 dried kaffir lime leaves (optional)*

Directions

In a medium bowl, combine Meatball ingredients and mix with your hands thoroughly. Make 28 meatballs by spooning heaping 1 tbsp of mixture and rolling between your hands. Lay on a cutting board or plate. Set aside.

In a small bowl, whisk together Sauce ingredients and set aside.

Preheat large ceramic non-stick skillet on medium-high heat and spray with cooking spray. Add meatballs and cook until brown or for 2-3 minutes, turning a few times. No need to cook the meatballs through.

Add the sauce, reduce heat to medium and simmer for 15 minutes, uncovered. Serve warm with brown rice or brown rice noodles. Add garnish like fresh cilantro and green onions.

Storage Instructions: Refrigerate covered for up to 3 days. Freeze in an airtight container for up to 3 months.

VEGGIE MAC AND CHEESE MUFFINS

INGREDIENTS

2 x 6 oz boxes Horizon Organic Mac and Cheese*

1/2 cup Horizon Organic milk or Silk almond milk

3 cups veggies, fresh or frozen

1 1/2 cups any Horizon Organic shredded cheese, divided

Cooking spray

Directions

In a medium pot, cook mac and cheese according to instructions on the box, undercooking pasta by 2 minutes.

Preheat oven to 350 degrees F. Line 2 muffin tins with parchment liners and spray inside with cooking spray. Set aside.

To a pot with cooked mac and cheese, add milk, vegetables and 1 cup of cheese. Mix well. Divide mixture evenly between 24 openings and sprinkle with remaining 1/2 cup cheese. Bake for 20 minutes.

Remove muffins from the oven and let cool in a tin for 30 minutes to allow muffins to set. Serve warm, hot or cold.

ONE POT CHICKEN AND BROCCOLI QUINOA

INGREDIENTS

Chicken:

2 lbs boneless & skinless chicken breasts, cut into 1" pieces

1 tbsp olive oil, extra virgin*

1/2 tsp cumin, ground

1/2 tsp all spice (optional but good)

1/2 tsphimalayan pink salt

Ground black pepper, to taste

Quinoa:

2 medium onions, diced

3 large garlic cloves, minced

1 large carrot, shredded

1 tsp olive oil, extra virgin

1 1/2 cups quinoa, uncooked

3 cups boiling water

3/4 tsphimalayan pink salt

1/2 tsp cumin, ground

2 bay leaves

1 lb broccoli, chopped

Directions

Preheat large deep skillet or a Dutch oven on medium-high heat. Add Chicken ingredients and sauté for 10 minutes, stirring occasionally. Drain liquid if necessary and cook until golden brown sides appear. Transfer to a bowl and set aside.

Add olive oil, onions, garlic, carrot and cook for 3-5 minutes, stirring occasionally. Add pre-cooked chicken, quinoa, water, remaining salt and cumin, and bay leaves; stir. Bring to a boil, cover, reduce heat to low and cook for 20 minutes.

Now it's time to add broccoli. At this point quinoa should be cooked al dente. Add broccoli, stir, cover and cook for 5 more minutes. Serve hot.

SAUSAGE QUINOA WITH POBLANOS

INGREDIENTS

1 cup quinoa, uncooked

7 oz any chicken sausage, casings removed

1 tbsp coconut oil or avocado oil

1 medium red onion, finely chopped

2 large red bell peppers, finely chopped

1 large green bell pepper, finely chopped

6 smaller poblanos, finely chopped

1 tsp cumin

1 tsp salt

1/2 tsp chili powder

3 lime wedges, squeezed

Directions

Cook quinoa as per package instructions. In the meanwhile, prepare vegetables.

Preheat large non-stick skillet on medium heat and add chicken sausage meat. Cook until cooked through and browned pieces appear, stirring and breaking into small pieces with spatula. Transfer to a large bowl or dish.

Return skillet to medium heat and swirl oil to coat. Add onions and saute until translucent, stirring occasionally. Add red, green and poblano peppers and cook for another 5 minutes or so, stirring occasionally. Peppers should be fragrant and golden brown sides appear on some.

Return sausage to the skillet and add cumin, salt and chili powder. Stir well, remove from heat and transfer to a previously used bowl or dish. Fluff quinoa with a fork, add to a bowl, squeeze lime on top and stir gently until well mixed. Serve hot or cold.

HEARTS OF PALM STRAWBERRY SUMMER SALAD

INGREDIENTS

3 cups baby lettuce

8 ounces fresh strawberries, stems removed and sliced

14 ounce can or jar of hearts of palm

1 small cucumber, cleaned and cubed

1 avocado, peel removed, cubed

1/2 cup strawberry lemon poppy seed dressing

INSTRUCTIONS

Divide lettuce between two bowls. Top with strawberries, hearts of palm, cucumber and avocado. Drizzle with the strawberry lemon poppy seed dressing.

CURRY CHICKEN SALAD WITHOUT MAYONNAISE

INGREDIENTS

1-1/2 pounds cooked chicken, cut into strips or cubes

1 cup cashew curry sauce

1/4 cup pecans, toasted and chopped

1/4 red grapes, quartered (optional)

1/4 cup celery, minced to similar sizes as the above

INSTRUCTIONS

Combine all of the aboveand allow the flavors to sit for a little while in the fridge before serving.

Serve on top of lettuce or apple slices for a gluten free, dairy free lunch.

VEGAN BROCCOLI SALAD WITH CASHEW CURRY DRESSING

INGREDIENTS

2 heads of broccoli, trimmed and cut into small florets

2 carrots

1/2 cup of raisins

Cashew Curry Dressing

3/4 cup raw cashews, soaked overnight in water

2 tablespoons apple cider vinegar

1 garlic clove

1 tablespoon maple syrup (or other sweetener of your choice)

1/2 teaspoon Dijon mustard

1/2 teaspoon Muchi Curry

2/3 cup of water

INSTRUCTIONS

Drain and rinse the cashews after they are soaked in water overnight. Place in a food processor or high speed blender, and add the remaining dressing ingredients, taking care to slowly add the water, adjusting more or less until it reaches your ideal consistency. It should be fluid enough to pour over your salad, but thick enough to stick to the florets.

Place the broccoli florets in a bowl and add enough dressing so it coats the broccoli. You won't need all of it. Then use a vegetable peeler to add strands of carrots to the salad. Toss with raisins and serve.

QUINOA AND VEGGIE FILLED TURKEY CUPS

INGREDIENTS

1 package natural turkey or 16 long, thin slices of leftover turkey

½ cup cooked quinoa

½ cup yellow squash, diced

½ cup zucchini, diced

16 cherry tomatoes, quartered

1 tablespoon shallots, minced

½ teaspoon dried basil

½ teaspoon dried thyme

Juice from ½ lemon

1 flax egg (1 tablespoon flax meal in 3 tablespoons water, rest 10 minutes)

Salt and pepper to taste

INSTRUCTIONS

Preheat oven to 350.

Place the quinoa, squash, zucchini, tomatoes, shallots, basil, thyme, lemon, flax egg and salt and pepper in a bowl and stir until combined. Put in the refrigerator while assembling the turkey cups.

Spray a muffin pan with non-stick cooking spray. Place a piece of turkey in each muffin hole, ensuring to cover the sides and bottom. You may need to trim the turkey so it fits. Once all the turkey slices are set, remove the quinoa bowl from the fridge and place a spoonful of the mixture in each tin, making sure not to overflow. Cook in the oven for 10-15 minutes or until turkey begins to brown and the cups are set.

Remove from oven and cool before eating.

WHITE BEAN TUNA CAKES

INGREDIENTS

1 tablespoon of chia seeds

15 ounce can white beans

2 - 5 ounce cans Bumble Bee Prime Fillet Albacore Tuna with Jalapenos & Olive Oil

2 tablespoons green onion, diced

3 tablespoons frech cilantro, de-stemmed and finely chopped

1/2 lemon - juice and zest

1/8 teaspoon celery salt

1/8 teaspoon garlic powder

INSTRUCTIONS

Preheat oven to 350.

Place the chia seeds in a small bowl and cover with 3 tablespoons of water and allow to sit in the refrigerator for 15 minutes.

Drain and rinse the white beans and place in a large glass bowl. Mash until the beans are broken, but still chunky. Add the tuna, green onions, cilantro, lemon, celery salt and garlic powder to the bowl and mix until combined. Once the chia "egg" is set, combine with the other ingredients.

Grease large muffin tins and evenly divide mixture into cups. Cook in the oven until set, approximately 20 minutes for 4" patties. Remove from oven and allow to cool on an oven rack.

Enjoy wrapped in a lettuce leaf and topped with avocado sauce

LIME CHICKEN TACOS WITH SPICY SLAW AND GUACAMOLE

INGREDIENTS

Spicy Slaw

2 tablespoons Dijon mustard

2 tablespoons fresh lime juice

2 garlic cloves, minced, about 1 teaspoon

1 tablespoon jalapeno pepper, minced

1/4 cup of apple cider vinegar

1/4 cup olive oil

2 small heads of cabbage - about 6 cups

3 carrots

Salt to taste

Chicken Marinade

4 tablespoons freshly squeeze lime juice

Zest of lime

1 tablespoon fresh ginger, minced

1/4 cup cilantro, stems removed, coarsely chopped

1 tablespoon canola oil

1.5 pounds of raw chicken breast

Guacamole

3 ripe avocados, peeled with seed removed

3 tablespoons fresh cilantro, stems removed, coarsely chopped

Juice of 1 lime

1 chipotle, diced with seeds removed

1/4 teaspoon celery salt

1/2 teaspoon Sriracha

8 small tortillas - gluten free or coconut paleo wraps

INSTRUCTIONS

- Prepare the slaw first so the flavors have time to set. In a large glass bowl, whisk together the Dijon, lime, garlic, jalapeno and vinegar. Slowly add in the olive oil.
- Place a grater attachment on a food processor and put the cabbage through in chunks. If you don't have a processor, cut the cabbage in quarters and then thinly slice so you have ribbons. Use a vegetable peeler to create carrot strands and add to the cabbage.
- Take the cabbage and carrots and combine them with the dressing and mix well. Salt and add additional lime if necessary. Allow flavors to rest and develop overnight or for a few hours.
- Place all the chicken marinade ingredients in a bowl and mix well. Pat the chicken dry and take a knife and score the skin in several places on both sides of the breast to allow the marinade to penetrate. Let the chicken sit in the marinade for 15 minutes or up to aa few hours in the refrigerator.
- Mash the avocados in a medium glass bowl. Fold in the rest of the guacamole ingredients. Mix well and set aside.
- Preheat oven to 350.
- Bring the chicken to room temperature when ready to cook, and place a grill pan over medium high heat. Once warm, add the chicken to the pan, cooking on both sides until opaque all the way through - approximately 10 minutes.

- Wrap the tortillas in tinfoil and place in the oven until warm. Layer the tortillas with the spicy slaw, grilled chicken and guacamole and enjoy

PINEAPPLE SHRIMP SALAD

INGREDIENTS

2 Zululand Queen baby pineapple

1 small English cucumber - diced

1/2 jalapeno (or to taste) - stem and seeds removed, finely chopped

1 avocado - peeled, cored and cubed

Juice of 1 lime

1/4 teaspoon of Sriracha

1/4 cup fresh cilantro, de-stemmed, and chopped

1 pound cooked shrimp

Salt and pepper to taste

INSTRUCTIONS

- Cut the pineapples down the middle. Take a paring knife and cut around the perimeter of the inside of the pineapple. Score the interior flesh into 4 blocks and then scoop out the inside.
- Take 1/4 cup of the pineapple flesh and muddle it (or use a mortar and pestle), creating a liquid juice. Chop the remaining pineapple flesh into small cubes.
- Add the shrimp, cucumber, jalapeno, avocado, lime, cilantro and Sriracha to the pineapple and mix. Season with salt and pepper. The flavors will develop the longer

you let it sit, but the lime juice will also continue to "cook" the shrimp so don't leave in the refrigerator more than a day.

- Scoop the mix back into the hollowed out pineapples and serve.

SALADE NIÇOISE

INGREDIENTS

1 medium shallot, minced

¼ cup fresh lemon juice (from approximately 2 lemons)

1 tablespoon Dijon mustard

1/3 cup olive oil

Salt and pepper

Optional: fresh herbs like basil, oregano, thyme, tarragon, parsley

SALAD

2 heads Boston or Bibb lettuce

1 pound green beans, French if possible

8 anchovies packed in olive oil

8 ounces canned albacore tuna in olive oil, look for BPA-free can

12 ounces cherry tomatoes, halved

½ cup black Niçoise olives

4 hard-boiled eggs, halved

INSTRUCTIONS

Place minced shallot, lemon juice and Dijon mustard in a bowl and whisk.

Slowly add the olive oil to the mixture until combined.

Season with salt and pepper and set aside.

Bring a large pot of salted water to a boil.

Trim the ends of the green beans.

Add the beans to the boiling water and cook for approximately 3 minutes, until tender but still crisp. Drain the beans and place them in a bowl filled with ice water to stop the cooking and keep them crisp.

Arrange the washed greens in a large bowl and dress with the vinaigrette.

Place each additional ingredient on top and drizzle the remainder of the vinaigrette. Salt and pepper as needed.

EASY BAKED LEMON CHICKEN

INGREDIENTS

¼ cup olive oil

3 tablespoons minced garlic (about 9 cloves)

? cup dry white wine

1 tablespoon grated lemon zest (about 2 lemons)

2 tablespoons freshly squeezed lemon juice

1½ teaspoons dried oregano

1 teaspoon minced fresh thyme

salt and pepper to taste

4 boneless chicken breasts

1 lemon

thyme sprigs for garnish

INSTRUCTIONS

- Preheat the oven to 400 degrees.
- Place the olive oil in a small saucepan over medium-low heat. Add the minced garlic and cook for just a minute. You want it to soften but not brown.
- Remove from the heat, and add the wine, lemon zest, lemon juice, oregano, thyme, and 1 teaspoon salt. Pour this mixture into a baking dish.
- Place the chicken breasts in the dish, and brush them with olive oil. Sprinkle with salt and pepper.
- Cut the lemon into wedges and place them around the chicken in the pan.
- Bake for 30 to 40 minutes, until the chicken reaches an internal temperature of 160 degrees. (If you use skin-on chicken, you can put it under the broiler for a couple minutes to brown the skin nicely. I didn't bother with the skinless.)
- Cover the pan tightly with aluminum foil, and allow the chicken to rest for 5-10 minutes. Garnish with thyme, and serve over rice with the pan juices. Add a salad or a steamed green vegetable for a complete dinner.

BAKED SALMON WITH LEMON CAPER BUTTER

INGREDIENTS

2 (5 ounce) salmon fillets

kosher salt and pepper

4 lemon slices

non-stick spray

LEMON CAPER BUTTER

3 tablespoons unsalted butter

2 cloves garlic, minced

2 tablespoons capers drained and rinsed

1/2 teaspoon lemon zest

juice of 1/2 of a lemon

kosher salt and fresh cracked pepper

INSTRUCTIONS

- Preheat oven to 450 degrees.
- Line a baking sheet with aluminum foil and spray with non-stick spray.
- Place salmon fillets on the prepared baking sheet.
- Sprinkle fillets with kosher salt and fresh cracked pepper. Place 2 lemon slices on top of each fillet. Bake for 10 minutes. Remove and tent with aluminum foil for 10 more minutes. Fish will continue to cook during this time. It will flake easily when done.
- While salmon is cooking, in a small sauce pan, melt butter over medium heat. Once butter has melted add garlic, capers, lemon zest and lemon juice. Cook for 2 minutes. Season to taste with salt and pepper.

- Remove lemon slices and discard. Gently slide a turner or serving spatula between the skin and the flesh of the fillet to remove the skin, it should separate very easily. Transfer fillet to a serving platter and spoon lemon caper butter over the top. Serve.

CHAPTER SIX
CLEAN EATING DINNER RECIPES

SIESTA TACO SOUP

INGREDIENTS

1 can fire-roasted diced tomatoes (28 oz.)

2 cups vegetable broth

1 can black beans, drained and rinsed

1 can kidney beans, drained and rinsed

1 can lentils, drained and rinsed

1 red onion, thinly sliced

2 cloves garlic, minced

1-2 fresh jalapenos

1 yellow bell pepper, diced into large pieces

2 tsp. chili powder

1 tsp. onion powder

2 tsp. Braggs soy sauce

2 1.2 tsp. cumin

1 tbsp. hot sauce

¼ tsp. paprika

1 tsp. oregano

¼ cup Diaya vegan cheddar, shredded

black olives, sliced

fresh cilantro, diced

½ cup quinoa (optional)

lean meat, chicken breast (optional)

Instructions:

Toss all ingredients (except Daiya cheddar, olives and cilantro into your faithful slow cooker and mix. Fire up your slow cooker to high and cook for 2 hours. Add salt and pepper, and perhaps more hot sauce, to taste. Cook for another hour. Serve with black olives, fresh cilantro and Diaya cheddar, and enjoy.

RATATOUILLE (SERVES 4-6)

INGREDIENTS

5 tomatoes, diced

1 zucchini, sliced

1 eggplant, sliced

1 green bell pepper, diced

1 onion, chopped

2 cloves garlic, chopped

3 tbsp. virgin olive oil

sea salt and pepper, to taste

1 cup water

fresh basil, sliced

Instructions:

Saute garlic and onions in olive oil. Add eggplant, zucchini and bell pepper for 8 minutes. Add tomatoes, basil, water, salt and pepper. Cook for just a few more minutes until vegetables are cooked but not too soft. Serve and enjoy.

SPICY LENTIL SLOPPY JOES

INGREDIENTS

1 cup lentils

4 cup water

2 onions

Cooking Spray

1 cup tomatoes, chopped

2 splashed apple cider vinegar

2 tbsp. mustard

Hot sauce or cayenne pepper

2 cloves garlic, minced

Pinch of ground sage

Pinch of cumin

Pinch of onion powder

Handful of fresh basil

Dash turmeric

Sea salt and pepper, to taste

1 cup tomato sauce

Romaine lettuce, chopped

Gluten-free bun (optional)

Instructions:

Boil lentils with water, cover until soft. Spray pan and sauté the onion, add tomatoes for 5 minutes. Add all ingredients to pan except for tomato sauce. Stir in lentils. Add tomato sauce, turn heat on medium for 10 minutes and stir often. Serve atop romaine lettuce or gluten-free bun, and enjoy.

SHEPHERDS PIE

INGREDIENTS

2 lbs ground beef

1 onion chopped

1 cup vegetables

2 lbs potatoes

8 tablespoons butter

½ cup beef broth

1 teaspoon Worcestershire sauce

Salt and pepper

INSTRUCTIONS

- Peel and quarter the potatoes, boil in salted water for 20-25 minutes or until tender.
- While the potatoes are cooking, melt a half stick of butter in a large frying pan and sauté onions, carrots and turnip in butter until tender.
- Add ground beef and sauté until no it's cooked thru.

- Add salt, pepper and Worcestershire sauce along with the beef broth and cook, uncovered, over low heat for 10 minutes.
- Mash the potatoes in bowl with another 4 TBSP butter, and season to taste.
- Place the beef mixture in a baking dish and spread mashed potatoes on top. Don't worry about making them smooth, some texture allows them to brown nicely.
- Cook at 400 degrees for 30 minutes, and serve hot.

LEMON-GARLIC SHRIMP SCAMPI WITH ZUCCHINI NOODLES

INGREDIENTS

3 Tablespoons olive oil

pinch crushed red pepper flakes

12 oz peeled and deveined shrimp

6 cloves garlic, minced

½ cup halved grape tomatoes

4 medium zucchini, spiralized

salt and pepper to taste

1 lemon, halved

INSTRUCTIONS

- Heat 2 tablespoons of the olive oil in a sauté over medium-high heat. Add the red pepper flakes and shrimp and a sprinkle of salt and pepper; cook for 2 or 3 minutes.

- Add the tomatoes and half the garlic; cook for one more minute, or until the shrimp is just cooked through. Set aside.
- Add the remaining tablespoon oil and garlic to the pan, give it a shake so the garlic starts to cook. Then add the zucchini noodles and another sprinkle of salt and pepper; cook for 2 or 3 minutes.
- Return the shrimp and tomatoes to the pan; squeeze the lemon over the dish. Serve immediately.

ROCKFISH WITH LEMON BUTTER & SAGE

INGREDIENTS

2 filets of rockfish

4 tablespoons butter

Old Bay Seasoning

1 lemon, sliced

Salt and pepper to taste

Sage, optional

INSTRUCTIONS

- Melt the butter in a casserole dish under the broiler.
- Sprinkle the rockfish filets lightly with Old Bay Seasoning, salt and pepper; add them to the casserole dish.
- Return the dish to the oven and broil the filets for 6-8 minutes, rotating halfway through.
- Remove from the oven and baste with the melted butter; place the lemon slices on top and sprinkle with sliced sage, if desired.

- Return to the oven long enough to char the lemon. Garnish with sage and serve hot.

PORK LOIN WITH LEEKS

INGREDIENTS

2 large leeks

¼ cup water

4 tablespoons butter, divided

1 teaspoon salt, divided

½ teaspoon black pepper, divided

1 (2-pound) boneless pork loin, trimmed

½ cup dry white wine

INSTRUCTIONS

- Remove roots and tough upper leaves from leeks and cut each in half lengthwise. Then slice them crosswise into ½-inch-thick slices. Soak in cold water to loosen dirt. I like to use a salad spinner.
- Combine leeks, ¼ cup water, 2 tablespoon2 butter, ½ teaspoon salt and ¼ teaspoon pepper in a large Dutch oven over medium-high heat. Cook for 10 minutes or until the leeks wilt, stirring occasionally. Pour them into a bowl.
- Heat the remaining 2 tablespoons butter the Dutch oven over medium heat and add the pork to pan. Cook 5 minutes, turning to brown on all sides. Add the remaining ½ teaspoon salt, remaining ¼ teaspoon pepper and wine to pan; cook 15 seconds, scraping pan to loosen browned bits. Return the leeks to the pan and

cover, reduce heat and simmer 2 hours or until the pork is tender.

- Remove pork from pan and cut into ¼-inch-thick slices. Spoon leeks over pork and serve.

BUTTERNUT SQUASH CLEAN EATING MACARONI & CHEESE RECIPE

INGREDIENTS

12 ounces Whole Wheat Elbow Macaroni Noodles

1 small Butternut Squash

2 Tbl Butter

2 Tbl Whole Wheat Flour

1 Cup Whole Milk

4 Cups grated Cheddar Cheese, divided

1/2 tsp Onion Powder

1/2 tsp Prepared Mustard

1/2 tsp Sea Salt + more to taste

1/8 tsp White Pepper

1/2 Cup Whole Wheat Bread Crumbs (use seasoned, if desired)

Instructions

- Cut or peel the skin off of the butternut squash, scrap out the seeds, and cut the squash into 1/2" cubes.
- Place in a saucepan and cover with water.
- Bring water to a boil. Reduce to a simmer and cook squash for 8-10 minutes, or until tender.

- Drain the water and place the squash in a food processor. Process until completely smooth. Set aside.
- Fill a large pot 3/4 full with water and season with 1/2 tablespoon salt.
- Bring to a boil. Add the macaroni noodles to the water.
- Stir once and let cook, stirring occasionally for 9-10 minutes, or until just under al dente. Pasta should be just a little firmer than you would want it to be when eating because it will continue to cook and soften in the oven when baking.
- Melt the butter in a large saucepan over medium/high heat.
- Whisk in the flour and cook for 30 seconds.
- Add 1/2 cup of the milk and whisk until thickened and smooth.
- Add in the butternut squash puree and whisk until smooth and bubbling.
- Add 2 cups of the grated cheese and whisk in until melted and smooth.
- Add the remaining 1/2 cup milk and whisk until smooth. Add 1 more cup of cheese and whisk until smooth.
- Add the onion powder, mustard, salt, and pepper, and whisk until smooth.
- Drain the cooked pasta and toss it with the cheese sauce.
- Scoop the pasta into a 9x13 pan. Sprinkle the remaining 1 cup of cheese on top.
- Sprinkle the breadcrumbs over the cheese and bake in an oven preheated to 400 degrees for 10-15 minutes or until hot and bubbling and cheese on top is melted.

CLEAN EATING SALMON RECIPE WITH A LEMON GARLIC HERB CRUST

INGREDIENTS

3 oz Organic Butter

1 tsp Coarse Real Salt

Zest of 1 Lemon

1 Tbl Fresh Parsley, chopped

1 tsp Fresh Dill, chopped

1 Clove Garlic, minced

Dash of White Pepper

4 4-5 oz Salmon Fillets

Instructions

- Place all ingredients except for salmon in a small bowl and melt in the microwave for 30-45 seconds.
- Stir until combined.
- Place the salmon fillets on a parchment lined baking sheet.
- Using a pastry brush, coat the salmon with the lemon herb butter, evenly spreading it over the tops of each fillet.
- Bake in an oven preheated to 400 degrees on the top or second to top rack for 10-12 minutes, or until salmon is cooked through and flakes easily with a fork.
- Alternately, the fish can be broiled on medium/high on the second to top rack for 8-10 minutes, or until cooked through. This method will give you a bit more crunchy, caramelized crust.

CHUNKY VEGETABLE AND ROASTED TOMATO MARINARA SAUCE RECIPE

INGREDIENTS

10 Roma Tomatoes, halved lengthwise

Real Salt and Pepper

Olive Oil, for drizzling

1/4 cup Olive Oil, divided

1 Sweet Onion, chopped

1 Yellow Bell Pepper, cut into small dice

2 Large Carrots, cut into small dice

1 1/2 tsp Coarse Real Salt

2 Sprigs Rosemary, chopped

1 tsp Oregano, chopped

Pinch Chili Flakes

2 Cloves Garlic, minced

1/2 Cup Water

2 Bay Leaves

Instructions

- Preheat the oven to 300 degrees.
- Place tomatoes cut side up on a baking sheet. sprinkle salt and pepper over the tops of the tomatoes and drizzle with a little olive oil.
- Roast in the preheated oven for 2 hours, until they are soft, fragrant, and browned on top.
- Remove from oven and let cool for 10 minutes.

- Place tomato halves, oil, and juices in a blender and pulse until roughly pureed. Set aside.
- Heat 2 tablespoons of olive oil in a large frying pan on medium/high heat.
- Add the onion, peppers, and carrots and saute for 4-5 minutes, or until the onion is translucent.
- Add the salt, rosemary, oregano, and chili flakes to the pan and saute for another 3-4 minutes. The vegetables should start lightly caramelizing.
- Add the garlic and saute for an additional 30 seconds.
- Add the water, bay leaves, and the roasted tomato sauce to the pan and reduce the heat to medium.
- Cover and let simmer for 20 minutes.
- Remove the bay leaves and adjust seasonings, adding more salt if desired.
- Serve over zucchini noodles.

SIMPLE CLEAN EATING CHICKEN KORMA RECIPE

INGREDIENTS

2 Tbl cooking oil of choice

6 large Chicken thighs, boneless and skinless

1 Yellow Onion, chopped

2 tsp .finely chopped fresh green chilies (serrano, Thai or jalepeno), optional

1 tsp Garlic, minced

Spices

1/2 tspGaram Masala

2 tsp Coriander

1/2 tsp Cumin

1/4 tsp Turmeric

1/4 tsp Cayenne, optional

Real salt and pepper, to taste

1 13-14 ounce can Coconut Milk, full fat

Last Minute Ingredients

1/2 Cup Cashews

1/4 Cup Shredded Coconut Flakes, unsweetened (optional)

Ginger Essential Oil, or alternately add 1/2 tsp ginger with the spices

Fresh Cilantro, to garnish

Instructions

Traditional Preparation

- Put all the main ingredients and spices in a oven-safe frying pan with high sides or an enameled dutch oven. Put the spices on both side of the chicken.
- Cook, turning the chicken half way through, until the chicken is 3/4th cooked, the onions are translucent and the spices are browned
- Pour the can of coconut milk into the pan and bring to a simmer. Cover.
- Place the pan in an oven preheated to 325 degrees. Cook for one hour, or until the chicken is tender.
- Shred chicken lightly. Check seasonings and add more salt, if desired. Add cashews, coconut flakes and ginger. Garnish with cilantro. Serve atop red quinoa or other grain, such as rice. Jasmine rice is my favorite, although

not strictly Clean Eating. I also really like short grain brown rice and mashed cauliflower with this dish.

GRILLED MAHI MAHI RECIPE IN A LEMON BUTTER SAUCE

INGREDIENTS

6 ounces MahiMahi fillets about 5-6 each

Real Salt and Pepper to taste

2 Tbl Olive Oil

6 Tbl softened Butter, divided (Ghee for Whole30 and possibly Paleo, depending on your beliefs)

1/4 small Sweet Onion minced

1/2 tsp Garlic minced

1/4 cup Chicken Stock

Juice of 2 small Lemons

Instructions

- Preheat a grill to medium/high heat.
- Place the MahiMahi fillets in a bowl and sprinkle salt and pepper over the top of the fish, to taste.
- Drizzle the olive oil over the fish and turn the fish to coat.
- Place the fish on the hot grill and let cook for about 3-4 minutes per side(depending on thickness), turning carefully.
- Remove from the grill to a serving dish.
- While the fish is cooking, melt 1 tablespoon of the butter over medium/high heat in a small saute pan.

- Add the minced onion to the butter and saute for about 2 minutes, or until softened.
- Add garlic and saute for an additional 30 seconds.
- Add the chicken stock to the pan and let simmer until reduced by half.
- Add the lemon juice and cook for 2 more minutes.
- Remove the pan from the heat.
- Add the remaining butter, 1 tablespoon at a time, to the sauce and stir in until the sauce thickens and becomes glossy.
- Add salt to taste, if desired.
- Pour butter sauce over the top of the grilled mahimahi and serve.

CLEAN EATING EASY SPANISH PAELLA RECIPE

INGREDIENTS

3 Tbl Olive Oil, divided

4 Chicken Thighs, Boneless and Skinless

Real Salt and Pepper, to taste

1 1/2 tsp Oregano, dried

14 ounce Turkey Sausage Link, sliced into 1/2" rounds, pre-cooked

1 Sweet Onion, sliced

2 Red Bell Peppers, sliced

3 Cloves Garlic, chopped

1/2 tsp Smoked Paprika

1 sprig Fresh Rosemary, chopped

15 ounce can Diced Tomatoes

2 Cups Short Grain Brown Rice

5 + Cups Chicken Broth

large pinch of Saffron

1 Cup Frozen Peas

8 Shrimp

8 Mussels, scrubbed

Instructions

- Heat 2 tablespoons of olive oil to medium/high in a large, deep frying pan. Season the chicken thighs on both sides with the salt, pepper, and dried oregano.
- Cook the thighs in the hot oil until golden brown on both sides. Remove chicken to a plate and cover.
- Add the sliced sausage to the same pan and broth the sausage slices on both sides. Remove the sausage and place with the chicken. Keep covered.
- Heat the chicken broth in a small saucepan, bringing to a boil. Remove from heat and add the saffron. Allow to infuse.
- In the same pan you cooked the chicken and sausage in, heat the remaining tablespoon of olive oil. Add the onion and bell pepper and saute until onion becomes translucent. Add the garlic, rosemary, and paprika and saute for another 30 seconds. Add the diced tomato and cook for another 2 minutes. Add in the rice and chicken broth. Bring to a simmer, reduce heat to medium and cover.
- Stir rice every few minutes. After about 35 minutes, start checking the rice for done-ness. If the liquid levels get too low, add a little more hot water or chicken broth to the

pan, 1/2 cup at a time. When the rice is almost tender, add the peas, mussels, and shrimp. Cook for another 3-4 minutes, or until mussels have opened and shrimp is bright pink.

- Taste and add more salt, if needed.

ORIENTAL CHICKEN SALAD RECIPE

INGREDIENTS

2 Large Chicken Breasts

Salt and Pepper, to taste

3 pieces smaller Romaine Lettuce Hearts, chopped into bite sized

1 Orange Bell Pepper, sliced (red or yellow would be fine too)

1 Large Carrot, peeled and sliced into very thin sticks

1/4 of a small Red Cabbage, shredded

15 ounce can Mandarin Oranges, drained

4 Green Onions thinly sliced

1/4 Cup Sliced Almonds lightly toasted

FOR THE DRESSING:

1/3 Cup Honey or Vegan sweetener of your choice

3 Tbl White Vinegar

2 Tbl Homemade Mayo

1 tsp Sesame oil

1/2 tsp Real Salt

Instructions

- Preheat the oven to 350 degrees. Place the chicken in a baking dish and season with salt and pepper. Bake in preheated oven for 25-35 minutes, until done. Cook time will really depend on the size of your chicken breasts. They should be at an internal temperature of 165 degrees when done. Remove chicken from oven and let cool completely.
- When the chicken is cool, cut into thin slices. In a large bowl, add the lettuce, bell pepper, carrot, cabbage, mandarin oranges, onions, almonds and sliced chicken.
- Whisk the honey, vinegar, mayo, sesame oil, and salt together in a small bowl. Pour over the salad ingredients and toss everything together.

SWEET POTATO CHICKEN SKILLET RECIPE

INGREDIENTS

2 Tbl Olive Oil

6 Chicken Thighs (boneless, skinless)

Coarse Real Salt (to taste)

Pepper (to taste)

1 Large Sweet Potato peeled and diced (1/2" cubes)

2 Carrots (peeled and cut into rounds)

1 Onion (cut into large slices)

3 Cloves Garlic (roughly chopped)

2 large sprigs Rosemary (chopped, stems removed)

1/2 tsp Cinnamon

1/4 tsp Allspice

1/2 tsp Coarse Real Salt

4 Tbl Honey

1/2 Lemon (juiced)

1/4 Cup Chicken Stock

1/4 Cup Toasted Almonds

1/4 Cup Dried Cranberries

Instructions

- Preheat the oven to 375 degrees.
- Heat the oil in a large frying pan to medium high. Season both sides of the chicken thighs with the coarse salt and pepper. Add the chicken to the hot pan and brown well on both sides. Remove the chicken from the pan and set aside.
- Add the sweet potato, carrots, and onion to the same pan the chicken was cooked in and saute until the vegetables develop some caramelization, about 5-6 minutes on medium/high heat. Add the garlic, rosemary, cinnamon, allspice, and salt, and saute for another minute. Add the chicken back into the pan and pile the vegetables over the tops of the chicken. Add the honey, lemon juice, and chicken broth to the pan and bring to a boil. Cover with an oven-proof lid and finish cooking in the oven for 35-40 minutes, or until chicken is tender. Remove the lid from the pan and cook an additional 5 minutes in the oven.
- Remove and garnish with toasted almonds and dried cranberries.

CROCK POT CHILI VERDE RECIPE

INGREDIENTS

2 lbs Tomatillos, husks removed

2 Poblano or Anaheim Peppers

2 Tbl Olive Oil

3 lb Pork Roast (Shoulder), cut into 1" cubes

2 Yellow Onions, cut into thick chunks

5 Cloves Garlic, chopped

1 tsp Oregano

1 Tbl Cumin

1/2 tsp Paprika

1/2 tsp Chili Powder

2 tsp Coarse Real Salt

1 Bunch Cilantro, bottom stems cut off

4 oz Can Green Chilis

2 1/2 C Chicken Broth

Lime wedges, to garnish

Avocado Slices, to garnish

Instructions

- Preheat oven to 450 degrees. Line a baking sheet with tin foil. Place the tomatillos(halve them if they are large) and the poblano or anaheim peppers on the lined baking sheet and place them on the top rack of the oven.
- Roast for 25-30 minutes, or until the tops are charred.

- While the tomatillos and peppers are roasting, heat the olive oil in a frying pan over high heat.
- Add the cubes of pork to the oil and brown on all sides. Place the pork in a slow cooker.
- Reduce the heat to medium/high and add the onion. Saute for 2 minutes, or until softened. Add the garlic, cumin, paprika, and salt and saute for another minute. Add the chicken broth, bring to a simmer and pour the mixture over the pork in the slow cooker.
- When the tomatillos and peppers have finished roasting, remove them from the oven. Remove the charred skin from the peppers and place them, and the tomatillos in a blender along with the cilantro and green chilis. Blend until smooth.
- Pour over the pork in the slow cooker.
- Cook on high for 4 hours or low for 6-8 hours.
- Check seasonings before serving and add more salt, if needed.

PISTACHIO CRUSTED CHICKEN STRIPS

INGREDIENTS

2 medium boneless chicken breasts

1 c unsalted, shelled pistachios

2 TBSP breadcrumbs

1 TBSP ground flaxseed

2 TBSP Dijon mustard

2 TBSP honey

1 TBSP coconut oil

Dipping Sauce (optional)

2 TBSP honey

2 TBSP Dijon mustard

Pre-heat oven to 350° F.

Line baking sheet with parchment paper.

In a small bowl, combine the mustard, honey and coconut oil. Mix well.

Finely chop pistachios either in food processor or blender.

In another small bowl, mix together ground pistachios, breadcrumbs and flaxseed.

Slice each chicken breast into three 1 inch long strips.

Dip each strip into mustard mixture to lightly coat, then roll through pistachio mixture until fully covered.

Place chicken strips on parchment paper baking sheet.

Bake chicken for 20 minutes, or until chicken is no longer pink and the outside is golden brown.

If you wish to dip the chicken in a honey mustard sauce, mix the two ingredients above while the chicken is cooking.

Serve over a large, fresh salad or with steamed veggies.

SALMON, SHRIMP AND TUNA SKEWERS

INGREDIENTS

6 oz skinless salmon steak, cut into 1/2-inch cubes (about 10 pieces)

6 oz skinless tuna steak, cut into 1/2-inch cubes (about 10 pieces)

10 medium peeled shrimp

1/4 cup extra-virgin olive oil

1 small lemon, juiced

2 garlic cloves, minced

1/2 cup chopped fresh flat-leaf parsley

1.5 TBSP coarsely chopped fresh thyme leaves

1/4 teaspoon freshly ground black pepper, plus extra for seasoning

Directions

- Whisk together olive oil, lemon juice, garlic, parsley and thyme for marinade.
- Place salmon, tuna and shrimp pieces in a gallon bag with marinade.
- Marinate in fridge for 30 minutes.
- Thread skewers with 2 pieces of each, rotating salmon, tuna and shrimp.
- Pre-heat a grill pan over medium-high heat or use a gas or charcoal grill.
- Season skewers with pepper to taste.
- Grill until opaque – 3-4 minutes on each side.
- Serve with grilled veggies and small side salad.

FOIL BAKED SALMON

INGREDIENTS

2 skinless salmon fillets (4oz each)

2 TBSP olive oil

2 tomatoes, chopped

1 TBSP fresh lemon juice

1/2 tsp dried thyme

1/2 tsp dried oregano

Ground black pepper and salt to taste

Directions

- Pre-heat oven to 400° F.
- Whisk together tomatoes, olive oil, lemon juice, thyme and oregano, then add the tomatoes and mix.
- Season salmon fillets with salt and pepper, drizzle one side with olive oil.
- Place single salmon fillet oiled side down on foil sheet.
- Wrap the ends of the foil to form a "boat". Do this for the second salmon fillet in a separate foil piece.
- Spoon tomato mixture evenly over both salmon fillets, covering them completely.
- Seal the foil boats completely closed.
- Place the sealed boats on a baking sheet.
- Bake about 25 minutes, or until cooked through.
- Remove salmon from foil boats and serve with red russet potatoes and green beans.

CHICKEN SALAD (NO MAYONNAISE)

INGREDIENTS

8 oz chicken breast, cooked, shredded (weighed, not in a measuring cup)

1 large avocado

2 TBSP olive oil

¼ c fresh basil leaves

½ tsp garlic

Ground black pepper and salt to taste

Directions

- In a food processor (or blender), mix together avocado, basil, olive oil, garlic, salt and pepper. Blend until creamy.
- In a medium bowl, stir together shredded chicken and avocado mixture until well blended.
- Season with extra garlic powder, pepper and salt as needed.
- Serve with whole wheat pita and small side salad.

CHAPTER SEVEN

CLEAN EATING SNACKS RECIPES

BROCCOLI TURMERIC FRITTERS - GLUTEN FREE, VEGAN

INGREDIENTS

1 tablespoon ground flaxseeds

2 cups broccoli

1/2 cup onion

1" fresh ginger

1" fresh turmeric

2 garlic cloves

1/4 cup cilantro

1/2 teaspoon ground curry

1/2 teaspoon ground cumin

1/2 cup chickpea flour

Salt to taste

1 tablespoon coconut oil (if not baking)

Hemp lime cream sauce for topping (optional)

INSTRUCTIONS

If baking, preheat the oven to 350.

Place ground flaxseed in a small bowl with 3 tablespoons water and set aside until set, about 10 minutes.

Trim the broccoli and pulse in the food processor until broken down without any large pieces. Remove the broccoli and place in a large glass bowl. Add the onion, ginger, turmeric, garlic, cilantro, curry and cumin to the food processor and blend. Add to the broccoli, along with the chickpea flour, flaxseed mixture and salt. Mix well with your hands until you achieve a nice dough. Adjust flour or add water until the mixture holds together well, but not too dry. Separate into 4 patties.

Line a baking sheet with parchment and bake the 4 patties for 30 minutes, flipping at the halfway point. Alternatively, you can cook on the stove top in coconut oil over low heat for about 20 minutes, flipping after 10 minutes.

CARROT PULP CUMIN CRACKERS

INGREDIENTS

1/2 cup carrot pulp

1/2 cup ground flax seeds

1/2 cup ground walnuts

2 tablespoons cumin seeds, ground

2 garlic cloves, grated

Salt to taste

INSTRUCTIONS

Preheat oven to 350.

Place all ingredients in a large bowl and mix with your hands until combined and you can form a ball. Separate equally into two halves.

Place one half in between two large pieces of parchment and pound out with your hand. Then take a rolling pin and roll the mixture until it's thin, but be careful not to tear. Transfer the rolled out piece to a parchment lined baking sheet and then repeat with the other half.

Bake in the oven for approximately 15-20 minutes, or until crisp. Check halfway through to ensure the ends don't burn. You can also score the crackers at this point, but I don't mind free flowing, random sized pieces. I also like to flip the cracker halfway through, but you need to be very gentle or it will break into many pieces. They'll turn into crackers anyway, so not a problem.

Enjoy out of the oven or keep on the counter in a tightly sealed container for 3 days.

GRANOLA CUPS WITH BANANA CREAM

INGREDIENTS

Granola Cups

1-1/2 cups gluten free rolled or old fashioned oats

1/4 cup ground flax meal

1 ripe banana, peeled and mashed

3 tablespoons coconut oil

3 tablespoons raw honey or agave nectar if vegan

1/2 cup toasted pecans, chopped

1/4 cup toasted almonds, chopped

Banana Cream

1 cup cashews, covered in water and soaked overnight

2 ripe bananas

1/2 teaspoon vanilla

1/2 teaspoon cinnamon

1 tablespoon raw honey or agave nectar if vegan

1/4 cup water

INSTRUCTIONS

Preheat oven to 350.

Place all granola cup ingredients in a bowl and mix until combined. Spray a muffin tin with non-stick spray and scoop a dollop of the granola mixture into each compartment. You should have enough mix to cover the bottom in a thin layer, as well as the sides. Wet your fingers to press down to form the cups, making them as thin as possible, but ensuring to cover all sides. Place in oven for 15-20 minutes, or until brown and crisp. Remove from oven and place the muffin tin on a wire rack and allow to cool before taking out the individual cups with a knife.

Place all of the banana cream items in a Vitamix or high speed blender and blend till smooth. Adjust the water accordingly. I prefer a thicker yogurt-like consistency.

Once the cups are cool, remove from the tin, top with banana cream and additional fresh fruit. Keep the additional cups in an air tight container in the refrigerator.

AVOCADO PESTO SALMON PINWHEELS {PALEO, GLUTEN FREE, DAIRY FREE}

INGREDIENTS

8 ounces of smoked salmon

2 ripe avocados, peeled with seed removed

1/4 cup pesto (use my kale pesto or spinach mint pesto)

INSTRUCTIONS

Take a piece of saran wrap and place it flat on a level surface. Lay pieces of salmon (about 4 ounces) side by side so it overlaps and makes one large piece (see picture above). Take one of the avocados and mash it so it's spreadable. Then spread the avo mash across the salmon, leaving room on each end for rolling. Top with half of the pesto. Start on one end and pull the wrap up and over to begin tightly rolling it. As you roll, move the saran on top and gently squeeze mixture together so it stay cohesive. When you get to the end, wrap the roll in the saran and refrigerate for a few hours or overnight to set (or slip in freezer for an hour). Repeat with remaining ingredients.

After it's set in the fridge or freezer, remove the wrap and slice into pieces. Enjoy immediately.

KALE ROSEMARY SUPER SEED CRACKERS

INGREDIENTS

1 cup kale chopped in the food processor, ribs removed

2 garlic cloves, minced

1 tablespoon rosemary, minced

1/2 cup ground flax

1/4 cup chia seeds

1/4 cup sesame seeds

1 tablespoon fresh lemon juice

1 tablespoon olive oil

Salt to taste

INSTRUCTIONS

- Preheat oven to 200 degrees Fahrenheit.
- Add all ingredients to a large glass bowl and mix with your hands until you form a ball. Place the ball between two sheets of parchment and roll out with a rolling pill as thin as possible, without breaking any of the edges.
- Put the rolled out dough on a baking sheet and use a pizza cutter to make scores in the crackers for later. Bake for about 45 minutes and then flip. Bake another 45 minutes or until crisp on both sides.

DELICIOUS CLEAN EATING HUMMUS

INGREDIENTS

3 cups cooked chickpeas (1 cup of dried)

¼ cup lemon juice

2 cloves of garlic

1/3 cup natural yogurt

1 sprig of rosemary

2 tablespoons of good quality avocado, safflower, walnut or extra virgin olive oil

Directions

Roast the garlic cloves in their skins to take the edge off. In a food processor blend together the chickpeas (if you can do this while they are still warm, they are easier to process), lemon juice, roasted garlic cloves, yogurt, rosemary leaves and oil until smooth. You can add a little salt and pepper to taste, but the aim is to add lots of fresh flavour and avoid needing salt to be able to enjoy it. If you love salt, try and adopt your palate to less salty tastes by adding only a small amount.

This dip should be enough for many snacks through the week when accompanied with carrot or celery sticks, which are easy to prepare and will happily last the week in the fridge when well covered and sealed.

FLOURLESS PUMPKIN BROWNIES

INGREDIENTS

1 cup pumpkin puree*

1/2 cup drippy almond butter (can sub for peanut, cashew or nut alternative spread)

1/4- 2/3 cup cocoa powder (more cocoa yields a richer taste)

Frosting of choice (optional)

Instructions

Preheat the oven to 350 degrees and coat a small 4 x 6 or 6 x 6 loaf pan with cooking spray and set aside- A smaller pan yields thicker brownies.

Add all your ingredients into a high speed blender, food processor or large bowl and mix until fully immersed and a thick batter is formed.

Transfer brownie batter to loaf pan and bake for 12-15 minutes, or until a skewer comes out just clean. Allow the brownies to cool in the pan completely before either frosting to slicing into bars.

PALEO PROTEIN BARS

INGREDIENTS

1 cup coconut flour, sifted

4 scoops flavored protein powder

1/2 cup + dairy free milk of choice*

1/2 cup smooth nut butter of choice (optional)

Dairy free chocolate chips (optional)

Instructions

Line a baking tray with baking paper, grease it and set aside.

In a large mixing bowl, combine the coconut flour and protein powder and mix well. If using the optional nut butter, add that in now.

Using a 1/4 cup at a time, at dairy free milk of choice until a very thick batter is formed. Transfer batter to lined baking dish and press firmly in place. Top with optional chocolate chips refrigerate for at least 30 minutes. Slice into bars and keep refrigerated.

FLOURLESS APPLE PIE BLONDIES

INGREDIENTS

1/2 cup unsweetened applesauce

1/2 cup almond or cashew butter (Can sub for peanut butter if not strictly paleo)

1/4 cup coconut flour, sifted

3-4 T pure maple syrup

1 T apple pie spice (a mixture of cinnamon, cardamom, nutmeg)

Optional- Coconut palm sugar + apple pie spice to top to form a small 'crust'

Instructions

Preheat the oven to 350 degrees and grease a baking tray

In a large mixing bowl, combine all the ingredients and mix very well until a very thick batter is formed. Transfer to the greased baking dish and bake in the oven for 30 minutes, or until the tops are golden. Remove from oven and allow to cool completely. Refrigerate for at least an hour before slicing.

NO BAKE COOKIE DOUGH PROTEIN BARS

INGREDIENTS

2 cups pitted Medjool dates

2 scoops vanilla protein powder

2-3 T chocolate chips

Instructions

Combine the dates and protein powder in a food processor.

Process until it just starts to clump together.

Stop and add the chocolate chips.

Continue processing until it forms one large ball of dough.

Shape into a rectangle. Cut into bars. Refrigerate overnight (or at least 4 hours)

Keep in the fridge.

BANANA CAKE COOKIES

INGREDIENTS

1/2 cup coconut flour, sifted

1/2 cup mashed banana (about 2 medium ones)

1/4 cup cashew butter

1/4 cup maple syrup

Dairy-free Chocolate chips (optional)

Instructions

Preheat the oven to 350 degrees and line a baking dish with baking paper and set aside.

In a mixing bowl, combine the coconut flour and banana and mix well- This should be very crumbly.

In a microwave safe bowl or stovetop, melt your nut butter with liquid sweetener and pour into the dry mixture. Mix until fully incorporated and a thick batter is formed. Add chocolate chips if desired.

Form into balls and transfer to the lined cookie sheet. Press firmly into a cookie shape and bake for 12 minutes. Remove and allow to sit for 10 minutes until they firm up slightly.

CLEAN EATING PROTEIN ICE CREAM RECIPE

INGREDIENTS

1 box Silken tofu

180g frozen berries

Optional: 1 scoop protein powder

Instructions

Place all ingredients in your blender or food processor and blend until smooth and creamy

Enjoy the clean eating ice cream straight away, or store in the fridge/freezer to have later

CLEAN EATING TUNA PATÉ

INGREDIENTS

1 tin of tuna in Springwater

40 gr of full fat Greek yogurt (or soya yogurt)

Juice from half lemon

¼ tsp garlic powder

Salt and pepper to taste

Optional chives to garnish

Instructions

Drain the tuna

Place all ingredients (except garnish) in food processor and process for around 2 minutes or until mixture has no lumps and makes a paste

Place the paté in the fridge, cover with cling fill and refrigerate for minimum 5 hours

Serve with crackers and or on a brown toast.

FENNEL CRISPS

INGREDIENTS

2 fennel bulbs

1 tbsp extra virgin olive oil

Pinch of Celtic sea salt

Method

1. Preheat oven to 180°C/160°C fan/gas mark 4. Trim the stalks and base off fennel. Cut bulb in half, peeling layers of leaves apart

2. Place leaves on a baking tray, drizzle on oil and sprinkle lightly with salt.

3. Bake in the oven for 25 minutes, turning a few times and removing any smaller leaves that cook quickly. Cool for 15 minutes before serving.

HEALTHY FRUIT AND NUT PARFAIT SNACK

INGREDIENTS

1/2 cup plain greek yogurt

1 tablespoon protein powder

1/2 cup cherries, pitted and halved

1/2 cup strawberries, sliced

1 tablespoon walnuts, chopped

Instructions

In a small bowl combine the protein powder and the greek yogurt, mix well.

Top with cherries, strawberries and walnuts.

HEALTHY SNACK BARS WITH CHOCOLATE, NUTS AND DATES

INGREDIENTS

– 2 cups of Medjool Dates, pitted and diced

– 1/2 cup of raw skinless almonds

– 2 cups of raw cashew

– 3/4 of organic dark cocoa powder

– Sea salt

– 3/4 cup of shredded coconut

– 2 tea spoons of real vanilla extract

– 3 table spoons of water

Directions:

1. Combine dates, nuts, cocoa powder, and sea salt in a food processor; and pulse all ingredients together until everything's mixed well and texture's coarse.

2. Add the shredded coconut and vanilla extract, pulse to mix.

3. Add a little water, pulse. Add a little more water, pulse. Repeat until content becomes moist.

4. Line an 8×8 baking pan with parchment paper. Scrape content from food processor into the pan, and press with your hands and then a rubber spatula.

5. Put pan inside a refrigerator and chill for an hour.

TORTILLA" CHIPS

Directions

Take 2 small 6-inch corn tortillas and cut them each into 6 pieces.

Place on a cookie sheet and spray with Pam. Then bake in the oven at 350 for 15 minutes or until crispy and lightly browned.

Please note: you can make a whole tray of them and then once cooled, place in a Ziploc baggie for consumption later on.

BAKED ZUCCHINI CHIPS

INGREDIENTS

Zucchinis (1 zucchini makes about a medium sized bowl and was the perfect snack size for 1 person/me!)

Olive Oil (or if you are strict paleo, melt down coconut oil and use that instead)

Salt, as desired

Paprika, as desired

Instructions

Preheat oven to 250°F.

Slice zucchinis very thinly, about as thin as you can cut it with a knife (don't use a mandolin slicer).

Throw the zucchinis in a mixing bowl and sprinkle oil, salt, and paprika in it. Mix it all together gently. Two things to take note here:

1) Make sure you don't put too much olive oil so that is soggy. If this happens, your zucchini chips will come out too soggy.

2) Make sure you don't put too much salt on there because the zucchini will shrink a considerable amount once it is baked.

Line a baking sheet with either aluminum foil or parchment paper

Place zucchinis on baking sheet without touching each other like so:

Bake for 30 minutes.

Take out zucchini chips and check on them flipped them over to make sure they were evenly cooked.

Bake for another 30 minutes or until crispy (could take up to 45 mins or more depending on how thin zucchinis were sliced and different ovens), but keep an eye on them because if they cook too long, they get over cooked.

When crispy, take them out and let them air and cool down for a couple of minutes before you eat them! Be sure to eat them within an hour or two because they will start losing their crispiness!

QUESO DIP AND HOMEMADE CHIPS

INGREDIENTS

4 cups of cauliflower florets

1/2 cup of broth or milk of your choice

2 cloves of garlic, minced

2 tsp of butter or olive oil

1 1/3 cups of freshly shredded sharp cheddar or cheddar jack cheese

1 can of diced tomatoes with green chilies, drained - mild, medium, or hot depending on your taste

1/2 tsp salt

chili powder (optional)

cumin (optional)

Homemade chips

Corn tortillas

Olive Oil Cooking Spray

Salt

Instructions

Place cauliflower florets in a large microwave-safe bowl with enough water to just cover the bottom of the bowl. Cover bowl loosely with waxed paper or a paper towel and steam cauliflower in microwave on high until tender, 4 to 5 minutes; drain.

Using a food processor, blend cauliflower with broth or milk to make a puree. Set aside.

Heat a skillet over medium-low heat. Melt butter and saute garlic 1-2 minutes or until fragrant. Add cauliflower puree to skillet and heat until warm, then stir in cheese until melted. Next add in drained tomatoes and salt. Cook on low ten minutes or until the flavors blend. Sprinkle in some chili pepper and cumin if desired, adjusting to taste.

Garnish with cilantro or jalapeno if you are feeling it!

For the chips - cut Corn tortillas into 6 pieces and lay them on a baking sheet lined with parchment paper. Spray with olive oil spray and cook for 8-10 minutes at 350. Chips will crisp up as they cool.

CHAPTER EIGHT

CLEANING EATING DESSERT RECIPES

GREEK YOGURT WITH ORANGES AND MINT

INGREDIENTS

6 tablespoons fat-free Greek yogurt

1 1/2 teaspoons honey

1 large orange, peeled, quartered and sliced crosswise

4 fresh mint leaves, thinly sliced

Directions

Stir together the yogurt and honey. Spoon yogurt mixture over the orange slices; scatter mint on top.

PINEAPPLE-COCONUT SORBET

INGREDIENTS

1/2 cup lite coconut milk

1/2 cup sugar

3 1/4 - inch slices peeled fresh ginger, crushed

1 pineapple, (about 3 1/2 pounds), peeled, cored and cut into chunks

2 teaspoons lime juice

Directions

Combine coconut milk, sugar and ginger in a small saucepan. Bring to a simmer over medium heat. Simmer for 1 1/2 minutes. Remove from heat and let stand for 20 minutes. Strain into a large bowl.

Place pineapple in a food processor and process until smooth. Add the pineapple puree to the coconut milk mixture and whisk until blended. Whisk in lime juice. Cover and refrigerate until chilled, about 1 hour.

Pour the pineapple mixture into an ice cream maker and freeze according to manufacturer's directions. (Alternatively, freeze mixture in a shallow metal pan until solid, about 6 hours. Break into chunks and process in a food processor until smooth.)

Serve immediately or transfer to a storage container and let harden in the freezer for 1 to 1 1/2 hours. Serve in chilled dishes.

CHOCOLATE-DIPPED BANANA POPS

INGREDIENTS

2 ounces roughly chopped unsweetened baking chocolate

3 ounces roughly chopped milk chocolate

2 ripe bananas

1/3 cup coarsely chopped salted peanuts (or toasted coconut or cacao nibs if desired)

Directions

Melt chocolate in a heat-proof bowl set over a pan of simmering water, stirring occasionally, until smooth. Meanwhile, line a baking sheet with parchment or wax paper. Slice bananas into thirds crosswise; insert a wooden freezer-pop stick or skewer in one end of each. Dip pieces in melted chocolate, spooning on additional chocolate to cover. Place on prepared baking sheet and sprinkle with chopped salted peanuts. Freeze until chocolate is firm, about 20 minutes, or up to 2 hours. (If frozen for more than 2 hours, let soften for 20 minutes before serving.)

BANANA WITH DARK CHOCOLATE-HONEY SAUCE

INGREDIENTS

2 tablespoons bittersweet chocolate chips or chopped dark chocolate

1 teaspoon honey

1 teaspoon unsalted butter

Small pinch of salt

1 small banana, peeled and cut into 1-inch chunks

1 teaspoon chopped toasted walnuts

Directions

In a double boiler or microwave-safe bowl, melt the chocolate with the honey, butter and salt, stirring frequently. Serve the chocolate sauce and walnuts in bowls for dipping, accompanied by the banana chunks.

MINI PALEO MAPLE CUPCAKES

INGREDIENTS

4 tablespoons (or ¼ cup) of Grass-Fed/Clarified Butter or Extra Virgin Coconut Oil

½ cup Unsweetened Applesauce

4 Eggs

1 teaspoon Vanilla Extract

4 teaspoons Maple Syrup

¾ cup Almond Flour

2 teaspoons Cinnamon

½ teaspoon Baking Powder

1/8 teaspoon Kosher Salt

CINNAMON MAPLE FROSTING

1 cup Palm Shortening

2/3 cup Maple Syrup or Honey

1 teaspoon Vanilla Extract

1 teaspoon Maple Flavoring

4 tablespoons (or ¼ cup) Arrowroot

2 teaspoons Coconut Flour

2 teaspoons Cinnamon

2 tablespoons Chilled Coconut Milk Cream

Topping:

½ Apple Thinly Sliced

Cinnamon for Dusting

Directions:

Apple Cakes:

Preheat oven to 350 degrees F. Line mini cupcake pan with 24 paper liners.

Melt the butter then whisk in with the applesauce, eggs, vanilla, and maple syrup.

Add the almond flour, cinnamon, baking powder, and salt to the wet ingredients and mix until evenly combined.

Evenly distribute into the 24 mini cupcake liners {about 1 tablespoon of batter each} and bake at 350 F for 18 – 19 minutes. The cakes are done when a toothpick can be poked in and come out without any batter on the stick.

Let the cool completely.

Cinnamon Maple Frosting:

Whisk the shortening, maple syrup, vanilla, maple extract, arrowroot, coconut flour, and cinnamon together until smooth.

Add the chilled coconut milk cream and whisk again until smooth.

Use immediately. Either spoon the frosting into a gallon plastic bag or a pastry bag.

Gently frost each cupcake with your desired amount of frosting.

Store the rest of the frosting in the refrigerator. Let it come to room temperature before you use as frosting again.

Topping:

Top each cupcake with a thin slice of fresh green apple and dust with ground cinnamon.

If you don't enjoy the cupcakes immediately, store them in an airtight container in the refrigerator.

CARROT CAKE OATMEAL COOKIES

INGREDIENTS

1 cup (100g) instant oats

¾ cup (90g) whole wheat

1 ½ tsp baking powder

1 ½ tsp ground cinnamon

salt

2 tbsp (28g) coconut oil or unsalted butter, melted and cooled slightly

1 large egg, room temperature

1 tsp vanilla extract

½ cup (120mL) pure maple syrup

¾ cup (68g) grated carrots (about 1 smallish medium)

In a medium bowl, whisk together the oats, flour, baking powder, cinnamon, and salt. In a separate bowl, whisk together the coconut oil, egg, and vanilla. Stir in the maple syrup until thoroughly incorporated. Add in the flour mixture, stirring just until incorporated. Fold in the carrots. Chill the dough for at least 30 minutes. (If chilling longer, cover with plastic wrap, ensuring it touches the entire surface of the cookie dough.)

Preheat the oven to 325°F, and line a baking sheet with a silicone baking mat or parchment paper.

Drop the cookie dough into 15 rounded scoops on the baking sheet. (If chilled longer than 1.5 hours, flatten slightly.) Bake at 325°F for 12-15 minutes. Cool on the baking sheet for at least 15 minutes before turning out onto a wire rack.

CHOCOLATE CARAMEL PEANUT BARS

INGREDIENTS

Caramel:

3/4 cup plain Greek yogurt

1 Tbsp oat flour

1/2 cup Xylitol

1/2 cup Xylitol Brown No Calorie Sweetener

1 tsp salt

1 tsp vanilla

1/2 cup dry-roasted unsalted peanuts

Filling:

1/2 Tbsp water + 1 Tbsp water

1/8 cup brown rice syrup

1 Tbsp coconut oil, melted

1/2 tsp vanilla (avoid HFCS)

1 Tbsp natural peanut butter

dash of salt

1.5 cups Stevia in the Raw

Coating:

8-10 ounces dark chocolate, melted

Directions:

1. Make the caramels:

In a medium sized saucepan, combine everything except for the vanilla and peanuts.

Bring to a boil over medium-high heat, stirring with a wooden spoon.

Reduce heat and continue to stir for approx 20 minutes. Add vanilla.

Once combined, place the mixture aside while making the rest of the bar.

Do NOT add the peanuts yet!

2. Using an electric mixer, combine 1/2 Tbsp water, brown rice syrup, melted coconut oil, vanilla, natural peanut butter, and salt until creamy. Slowly add Stevia in the Raw. Note: The Stevia in the Raw gives it a somewhat bitter taste at this point - this is okay!

3. Once combined, remove it from the bowl with your hands and press it into a lined or greased 4" pan. Place in refrigerator to cool.

4. If your caramel has hardened, heat it back up for a few minutes until soft. Once soft, mix in the peanuts. Once filling from step 3 is firm, pour caramel over the filling. Place back in refrigerator to cool.

5. Once your refrigerated mixture is firm (this could take a few hours), melt the chocolate in the microwave for approx. 2 minutes, stirring halfway through. Cut mixture into bite size bars and dip in melted chocolate to cover, using a fork.

6. Place bite size bars onto wax paper and allow to cool (this could take a few hours).

CHOCOLATE AVOCADO PUDDING

INGREDIENTS

2 avocados

1 scoop/packet of TLS vanilla whey protein powder

1 cup unsweetened almond milk

2 Tbsp chia seeds

1.5 Tbsp cocoa powder

6 small scoops stevia

pinch sea salt

Directions:

1. Add all ingredients to a Vitamix and blend until desired consistency is reached.

2. Place in refrigerator for 30 minutes to one hour or until chilled.

3. Enjoy!

CHOCOLATE APPLE OATMEAL PROTEIN BARS

INGREDIENTS

2 cups rolled oats

1/2 cup natural nut butter

1 tbsp coconut oil

1 tbsp ground flaxseed

4 scoops chocolate protein powder

3/4 cup unsweetened applesauce

Directions:

1. Line an 8" square baking dish/pan with parchment paper (wax paper will also work if you do not have parchment paper on hand).

2. Warm the nut butter and the coconut oil in the microwave for 15-20 seconds to soften.

3. Combine all ingredients in a medium-sized bowl. Mix using hands or a spoon until well blended.

4. Pour mixture into lined dish and smooth with the back of a spoon until even.

5. Place in freezer for 45 minutes. Remove from freezer, lifting parchment paper and bars out of the pan and place on a flat surface. Using a pizza wheel, cut into 8 bars. Serve.

CHOCOLATE ALMOND BISCOTTI

INGREDIENTS

1/2 cup raw unsalted whole almonds, toasted and coarsely chopped, divided (can also use chopped, unsalted almonds in bags from the grocery store)

1/2 cup unbleached all-purpose flour

1/3 cup whole wheat flour

1/2 cup unsweetened dark cocoa powder

2 tsp instant coffee crystals

1/2 tsp baking soda

1/8 tsp sea salt

1/2 cup Sucanat or rapadura sugar

1 whole egg

1 egg white

1 tsp real, high quality, vanilla extract (no HFCS)

1 tsp almond extract

1 tsp lemon zest

Directions:

1. Preheat oven to 350 degrees F/ 180 degrees C.

2. Line a baking sheet with parchment paper (optional)

3. Put 1/4 c of the almonds, both flours, cocoa powder, coffee crystals, baking soda and salt in a food processor. Process for a few minutes until the almonds are finely ground. Put mixture in large mixing bowl and set aside.

4. Combine Sucanat, egg, egg white, both extracts and lemon zest in a blender and process until mixture is foamy - three to four minutes.

5. Pour wet ingredients into flour mixture. Add remaining coarsely chopped almonds. Mix well.

6. Divide dough in two. Shape each half into a log and place logs on baking sheet.

7. Place baking sheet in the oven and bake for 15 minutes. Remove from oven and let cool for at least 10 minutes. Reduce heat to 300 degrees F/ 148 degrees C.

8. Cut each log into ten 1/2 inch pieces. You may choose to cut diagonally or straight.

9. Return the biscotti slices to the baking sheet and bake for 20 minutes or until the cookies are dry and lightly browned.

10. Remove from heat and place on wire rack to cool. Do not seal in airtight container until biscotti are cool and dry

PEANUT BUTTER BALLS

INGREDIENTS

1/2 cup natural peanut butter

2 Tbsp honey

5/8 cup dark chocolate, broken into pieces

1 1/4 tsp coconut oil

Directions:

1. Mix peanut butter and honey together using an electric mixer until thick (approx 1 minute).

2. Roll into balls and freeze for at least 45 minutes.

3. Combine chocolate chips and coconut oil and heat in microwave for 1 minute. Stir. Heat in microwave for another minute (or until melted).

4. Let chocolate/coconut oil mixture sit out for approx 10 minutes to slightly harden.

5. Once balls are chilled, dip in chocolate mixture.

6. Place balls into the refrigerator to chill.

HONEY GLAZED BANANAS

INGREDIENTS

1 large banana

2 tsp honey

1/2 tsp cinnamon

Directions:

1. Slice banana into 1/4-1/2" slices

2. Combine honey & cinnamon into small bowl (if necessary, heat honey in microwave until it is liquid enough to spread over bananas)

2. Spray pan using an olive oil mister

3. Once pan is warm, add banana slices

4. Cook on one side until browned (1-1 1/2 minutes) then flip over & cook (1-1 1/2 minutes)

5. Add honey & cinnamon mixture over banana slices

6. Flip bananas back over one more time for a few seconds & then serve

CHOCOLATE WHOOPIE PIES

For the Whoopie Cookie

INGREDIENTS

5/8 c dark, unsweetened cocoa powder

1/2 c oat flour

1/4 c coconut flour

1/8 tsp salt

1 c Stevia in the Raw

1/2 tsp baking soda

1/8 tsp baking powder

2/3 c unsweetened applesauce

1/2 tsp vanilla extract (avoid HFCS)

1 egg

Directions:

1. Preheat oven to 325 degrees F. Mix together dry ingredients in a bowl, whisking to combine. Mix wet ingredients in a bowl, combining thoroughly with a whisk, handheld mixer or a stand mixer.

2. Slowly incorporate dry ingredients into wet ingredient mixture, whisking to combine. Your batter will be of a dough-like consistency and very sticky.

3. Line a baking sheet with parchment paper OR use a non-stick baking sheet lightly spritzed with olive oil. Using a spoon, drop small dough balls onto a baking sheet.

4. Bake for approximately 15 minutes.

STRAW-NANA-NUT ICE CREAM

INGREDIENTS

2 frozen Bananas

6 oz Organic Strawberries

1/2 cup of raw whole Cashews

Directions:

1. Soak cashews in warm water at room temperature for 2-12 hours. Drain cashews once they have been soaked.

2. Dice organic strawberries.

3. Slice frozen bananas into 1/4" slices.

4. Puree strawberries & cashews in a Vitamix until smooth (start at the lowest speed & gradually turn it up to 4). Add up to a 1/4 cup of water, if needed. Add bananas & puree again, until very smooth.

5. Freeze in a sealed freezer proof container until just solid, approx 4 hours.

SAUTEED CINNAMON APPLES

INGREDIENTS

Organic Apple(s)

Coconut Oil (to coat the pan)

Cinnamon

Directions:

1. Wash and chop apple into desired size

2. Lightly coat pan with coconut oil, just enough to cover (less than 1/2 tsp)

3. Heat coconut oil in pan, once hot add apples

4. Sprinkle apples with cinnamon and stir until desired texture is reached

PUMPKIN PROTEIN COOKIES

INGREDIENTS

2 heaping Tbsp almond butter or natural peanut butter

1 heaping Tbsp pumpkin

3 Tbsp gluten free quick cooking oats

2 scoops vanilla whey protein

2 Tbsp Xylitol

1 oz egg whites (1-2 egg whites)

1/4 tsp baking soda

Directions:

1. Using a whisk or fork, mix all ingredients.

2. Bake at 350 degrees for 6 minutes.

SWEET POTATO AND CINNAMON BROWNIE

INGREDIENTS

1 cup Whole Wheat Flour (Substitute gluten free flour, such as Gluten-Free Oat Flour)

1 cup Unsweetened Cocoa Powder

1 Tbsp Ground Cinnamon

1 Tbsp Baking Powder

1/4 tsp Sea Salt

1 cup Baked Sweet Potato (Make sure that you use oven baked sweet potato minus the skin for maximum sweetness.)

1/2 cup Agave Nectar

1/4 cup Olive Oil

1 tsp Pure Vanilla Extract (no HFCS)

6 Egg Whites

Extra Olive Oil in a Spritzer Bottle

Directions:

1. Preheat Oven to 350 degrees F.

2. Combine flour, cocoa powder, cinnamon, baking powder and salt in a medium bowl. Set aside.

3. Using a food processor, combine baked sweet potato, agave nectar, oil and vanilla extract. Puree until combined and smooth.

4. Gradually mix wet ingredients into dry ingredients, until just combined.

5. In a separate bowl, whisk egg whites until fluffy.

CLEAN SWEET-BUT-TART GUMMIES

INGREDIENTS

3/4 c Fresh Squeezed Lime Juice (Approximately 8-10 limes depending upon size)

3 TBSP Local Raw Honey

3.5 TBSP Agar Powder

1/3 c Stevia in the Raw

Directions:

1. Combine lime juice, local honey and agar powder in a small sauce pan. Whisk to combine on low heat.

2. Once combined, remove from heat (this should only take a minute or two).

3. Pour in a square baking pan and place in refrigerator for approximately 2 hours.

4. Remove gummies from pan and slice into 1"x1" cubes.

5. Roll cubes in stevia for added sweetness.

THE BANANA SPRINT

INGREDIENTS

1 banana

1/4 cup Greek yogurt

1 scoop chocolate protein powder

1 tsp unsweetened vanilla almond milk or water

Optional Toppings:

1 tsp almond butter

1/4 cup oats

Directions:

1. Peel and cut banana in half, length-wise

2. Mix together Greek yogurt, protein powder, and almond milk

3. Add Greek yogurt mixture to open banana

33596615R00077

Made in the USA
Middletown, DE
16 January 2019